Manual of Panic-Focused Psychodynamic Psychotherapy

Barbara L. Milrod, M.D.
Assistant Professor of Psychiatry
Cornell University Medical College
Member, New York Psychoanalytic Society
New York, New York

Frederic N. Busch, M.D.
Instructor of Psychiatry
Cornell University Medical College
Faculty Member
Columbia University Center for
Psychoanalytic Training and Research
New York, New York

Arnold M. Cooper, M.D.
Professor Emeritus of Consultation-Liaison Psychiatry
Cornell University Medical College
Training and Supervising Psychoanalyst
Columbia University Center for
Psychoanalytic Training and Research
New York, New York

Theodore Shapiro, M.D.
Professor of Psychiatry in Pediatrics
Cornell University Medical College
Training and Supervising Psychoanalyst
The New York Psychoanalytic Institute
New York, New York

American Psychiatric Press, Inc.

Washington, DC
London, England

Note: The authors have worked to ensure that all information in this book concerning drug dosages, schedules, and routes of administration is accurate as of the time of publication and consistent with standards set by the U.S. Food and Drug Administration and the general medical community. As medical research and practice advance, however, therapeutic standards may change. For this reason and because human and mechanical errors sometimes occur, we recommend that readers follow the advice of a physician who is directly involved in their care or the care of a member of their family.

00 99 98 97 4 3 2 1

American Psychiatric Press, Inc.
1400 K Street, N.W., Washington, DC 20005

Library of Congress Cataloging-in-Publication Data
Manual of panic-focused psychodynamic psychotherapy / by Barbara Milrod . . . [et al.].
p. cm.
Includes bibliographical references and index.
ISBN 0-88048-871-9 (alk. paper)
1. Panic disorders—Treatment. 2. Psychodynamic psychotherapy. I. Milrod, Barbara.
[DNLM: 1. Panic Disorder—therapy. 2. Agoraphobia—therapy. 3. Psychotherapy—methods. WM 172 M294 1997]
RC535.M36 1997
616.85'2230651—dc20
DNLM/DLC 95-41407
for Libray of Congress CIP

British Library Cataloguing in Publication Data
A CIP record is available from the British Library.

Contents

Chapter 1
Introduction

The syndrome we now call *panic disorder* was described initially by Freud (1895/1962). Freud labeled this syndrome *anxiety neurosis;* his description included many of the characteristic traits that panic patients exhibit. He suggested that anxiety neurosis had a somatic—rather than psychological—etiology, related to particular sexual practices. In *Inhibitions, Symptoms and Anxiety* (Freud 1926/1950), Freud postulated that anxiety alerted the ego to the danger of emerging forbidden wishes. This anxiety could act as a signal, triggering the ego to use a variety of defense mechanisms to avoid the danger. Freud hypothesized that symptoms would arise from a compromise between the wishful impulse and the defense mechanisms elicited by the wish.

After Freud's new formulation, anxiety took on a central role in the psychoanalytic conceptual framework regarding the genesis of neurotic symptoms and character traits. However, the literature rarely distinguished between formulations for anxiety and those for anxiety attacks or panic disorder.

DSM-IV (American Psychiatric Association 1994) provides the current definition of panic disorder and agoraphobia. Panic disorder consists of recurrent panic attacks (discrete periods of intense fear or discomfort) accompanied by at least 1 month of behavioral change or persistent concern or worry about the attacks. Panic disorder often is accompanied by agoraphobia—the fear of entering situations or places from which escape may be difficult and in which the individual fears developing an embarrassing symptom or panic attack. Agoraphobia typically causes an individual to restrict his or her travel or activities.

The description of panic disorder and agoraphobia in DSM-IV derives in part from a trend toward the splitting of syndromes into increasingly discrete categories. This description contrasts with that of anxiety neurosis as Freud (1895/1962) described it, which contains a broader range of symptomatology and characterological issues—in addition to panic attacks—that psychiatrists now would regard as comorbid disorders.

DSM-IV differentiates Axis I syndromes primarily on the basis of specific symptom profiles and temporal criteria. This taxonomy has helped investigators in the development of systematic symptomatic research and helped them to determine the efficacy of treatment approaches to specific psychiatric syndromes. Yet some researchers and clinicians have criticized this approach for encouraging the separation of syndromes into what may be artificially discrete categories with limited clinical relevance; hence, they argue, the increasing recognition of comorbidity (Andrews et al. 1990; Tyrer 1985, 1986; Tyrer et al. 1992).

Research on treatment strategies for patients with panic disorder and agoraphobia has focused on the elimination of the frequent panic attacks and avoidant behavior that persons with this disorder exhibit. Researchers have reported high initial success rates with pharmacological and cognitive-behavioral therapeutic approaches in the treatment of these patients, although these patients frequently require continued treatment (Ballenger 1991; Noyes et al. 1989a, 1989b, 1990; O'Sullivan and Marks 1991). These studies show high rates of relapse and continued impaired global function with persistent anxiety symptoms in many patients following treatments that initially produce symptom relief (Fyer et al. 1987; Katon et al. 1992; O'Sullivan and Marks 1991; Pecknold et al. 1988). Furthermore, some patients cannot tolerate or do not respond to these treatments (Milrod and Shear 1991a, 1991b; Noyes et al. 1989a, 1989b; Rosenbaum 1992). These treatments have focused primarily on panic disorder and agoraphobic symptoms; they have not addressed the related psychosocial and psychological difficulties commonly found in panic patients (Katon et al. 1992; Markowitz et al. 1989).

The limited number of long-term follow-up studies of patients who have received psychopharmacological and cognitive-behavioral treatments for panic disorder have highlighted several problems and their limitations are reviewed in more detail by Milrod and Busch (in press). For example, investigators have found high rates of relapse—70%–90%—after discontinuation of medication (Fyer et al. 1987; Noyes et al. 1989a; Pecknold et al. 1988). Although cognitive-behavioral treatments claim lower relapse rates (Beck et al. 1992; Craske et al. 1991; Ost 1988), these therapeutic claims often are difficult to prove because patients are involved routinely in other, concurrent treatments. Moreover, patients often show only limited improvement in their panic and avoidance symptoms, rather than recovery. In summary, the limited number of follow-up studies suggest that most patients with this diagnosis continue to display symptoms and require further intervention.

This incomplete response by patients with panic disorder and agoraphobia may relate in part to the use of treatment strategies that consider these symptoms separately from the individual's personality. In a departure from the DSM-IV scheme, some clinicians and researchers have advocated regarding these patients as having a neurosis, which can include additional anxiety and depressive symptoms, as well as characterological problems (Andrews et al. 1990; Tyrer 1985, 1986; Tyrer et al. 1992). This approach is consistent with Freud's conception of anxiety neurosis (Freud 1895/1962), in which he included a wide range of accompanying symptoms and characterological predispositions. In this view, although panic attacks and agoraphobia are important features of the illness, more global characterological problems remain, leaving the individual vulnerable to recurrence.

Research suggests that patients with panic and agoraphobia appear to have a particular psychological predisposition that makes them vulnerable to panic onset and its potential recurrence (Klein 1964; Kleiner and Marshall 1987; Marks 1970; Torgerson 1986). Kleiner and Marshall (1987) suggested that "agoraphobia is rarely an isolated set of fears which exists in an otherwise well-functioning person" (p. 313). These patients often have personality disturbances, relationship problems, difficulties tolerating and defining inner emotional experiences, and unconscious conflicts about separation, anger, and sexuality. Cognitive-behavioral and pharmacological treatments do not focus on these areas of dysfunction.

Purpose of this Manual

Among available treatments, psychodynamic psychotherapy—because of its focus on intrapsychic conflict and characterological makeup—is well suited, in our view, to address the complexity of factors involved in panic vulnerability. Although researchers have not conducted systematic studies of the efficacy of psychodynamic treatment of panic attacks, the literature contains many case reports that describe successful treatment of panic disorder with psychoanalysis or psychodynamic psychotherapy (Abend 1989; Malan 1979; Mann 1973; Milrod 1995; Milrod and Shear 1991a, 1991b; A. M. Sandler 1988; Sifneos 1972; Silber 1989).

Milrod and Shear (1991a), for example, found 35 cases in the literature involving patients with well-described DSM-III-R (American Psychiatric Association 1987) panic disorder who had been successfully treated with psychodynamic psychotherapy or psychoanalysis. Information about the duration of treatment was available for 17 of these 35 patients. Of these 17 patients, 13 were treated for less than 4 months, 2 patients were treated in therapies described as "long-term," and the other 2 underwent what the reports described as "brief" treatment. These reports suggest that dynamic mechanisms may be operative factors in symptom formation and that this treatment can bring relief—often as rapidly as psychopharmacological or cognitive-behavior therapy.

In this book, we catalog psychological factors that are common among panic disorder patients and describe how psychiatrists can address these factors within psychodynamic psychotherapy. Our primary purpose is to help clinicians working with patients with panic disorder and agoraphobia to develop additional therapeutic strategies. A subsidiary purpose is to provide a standardized approach to psychodynamic psychotherapy for patients with panic disorder; this standardization may facilitate systematic research on the efficacy of this treatment of panic disorder and agoraphobia.

Throughout this book, we present clinical examples involving patients who participated in psychodynamic treatment for panic disorder; these examples represent a sample of such patients that we have treated. We describe 32 cases in some form, involving patients ranging in age from 11 years through their mid-60s; approximately 60% were women. Most had exhibited panic disorder for more than 3 years (ranging from 1 month to 11 years), and many had been in treatment for panic before coming to one of us. Of these 32 patients, 6 did not have any degree of agoraphobia; 8 had some affective symptoms (dysthymic disorder or major depression) in addition to their panic disorder.

Psychodynamic Background

We derive our psychodynamic formulation of panic disorder from research and clinical observations of psychological factors in panic disorder, including life events preceding panic onset, premorbid personality traits, and assessments of patients' perceptions of their parents. Many studies suggest that panic onset frequently occurs immediately following significant acute stressors (Faravelli 1985; Last et al. 1984; Roy-Byrne et al. 1986; Solyom et al. 1974). Life events preceding panic onset include real or fantasized loss or rejection as well as change that demands more independent behavior from the patient. Common examples include job or location changes, graduation, marriage, and births.

Wade et al. (1993) carefully assessed agoraphobic patients with panic attacks for the presence of chronic stressors and treatment responsiveness. They found that 43% of patients described chronic stressors of marked to moderate severity as primarily marital and relationship difficulties. These patients demonstrated persistence of moderate to severe symptoms after completion of treatment, compared with patients who did not report stressors. The authors suggested that adjunctive interventions directed at helping patients develop more effective means of problem solving and coping with chronic stress may be essential for persons with agoraphobia who also are experiencing enduring life stressors.

Certain individuals are vulnerable to life events that trigger a panic state. Cognitive-behavioral theory describes catastrophic misinterpretation of life events to explain how stressors trigger panic (Craske 1988). In our view, the meaning of the event to the individual—conscious and unconscious—and affective symptoms triggered in response to the event play central roles in the development of panic attacks. Our focus on meaning is consonant with the idea of catastrophic misinterpretation; in our formulation, however, we consider unconscious configurations as well.

Personality traits predispose individuals to the onset of panic in the context of particular life stressors. Marks (1970), reported that the majority of agoraphobic patients had been "variously described as 'soft,' anxious, shy and dependent" before the onset of panic disorder (p. 541). Klein (1964) determined that half of the patients in his early study "seem to have suffered from a chronically high separation anxiety level throughout life and to have developed panic attacks under conditions where they were peculiarly vulnerable" (pp. 405–406).

Although researchers typically have assessed observations of premorbid personality traits of panic and agoraphobic patients retrospectively, some studies have attempted to assess these factors more systematically. Kleiner and Marshall (1987), for example, used a structured interview to carefully assess premorbid traits before the onset of agoraphobia with panic attacks. They found that patients reported a "history of dependence associated with unassertiveness" and described themselves as "highly socially anxious, and as being fearful of negative evaluations"; patients also demonstrated "difficulties in coping with anger and criticism and a tendency to comply with others" (Kleiner and Marshall 1987, p. 318 and pp. 318–319). In a study of adult patients with anxiety disorders, Torgerson (1986) found a significantly higher rate of reported chronic anxiety in the childhood histories of a panic disorder group compared with a group of patients with generalized anxiety disorder.

Psychological predisposition to panic can include the presence of particular perceptions of parents, as reported by panic patients. In a study of 100 phobic patients, for example, Tucker (1956) described patient reports of a "lack of parental affection, overprotection and overcriticism by parents . . ." (p. 827) in 77 cases; this study included no control group, however.

More systematic studies have provided further evidence of this phenomenon. Using the Parental Bonding Instrument (Parker et al. 1979)—a questionnaire found to be reliable and valid—Parker (1979) reported that a group of patients with social phobia and agoraphobia described their parents as having been significantly less caring and more controlling compared with how individuals without any known psychiatric disorder described their parents; Silove (1986) corroborated these findings in a group of agoraphobic patients compared with a group of people without psychiatric disorders. Using a different questionnaire that assessed perceptions of parents—the Egna Minnen Betraffande Uppfostran (EMBU) (Perris et al. 1980)—Arrindell et al. (1983) found that agoraphobic patients described their parents as having significantly less emotional warmth compared with nonagoraphobic control subjects' characterizations of their parents. In addition, agoraphobic patients viewed their mothers—but not their fathers—as being more rejecting compared with the control subjects' descriptions of their parents.

Thus, the evidence indicates that certain individuals are psychologically predisposed to the onset of panic in the context of particular life stresses. In Chapter 2, we explore these factors further and formulate a psychodynamic model to elucidate the psychological vulnerability to panic.

Chapter 2

A Psychodynamic Formulation for Panic Disorder

A pilot study was conducted at Payne Whitney Clinic to gain further information about the role of predisposing psychological factors in vulnerability to panic, as well as meaningful life events connected to panic onset (Busch et al. 1991). Senior training analysts (A.M.C. and T.S.) conducted psychodynamic interviews with nine consecutive patients who met DSM-III-R (American Psychiatric Association 1987) criteria for panic disorder who presented to the anxiety disorders clinic for treatment. A research psychiatrist/psychoanalytic candidate (F.N.B.) then reviewed the videotapes, assessing a number of factors including life events preceding panic onset, capacity to tolerate anger, conflicts about sexuality, descriptions of parents, and behaviors and attitudes other than panic disorder symptoms.

Identifiable, psychologically meaningful stressors preceded the onset of panic in all of the patients evaluated in this manner. Furthermore, all of the stressors involved a loss or an alteration in the level of expectations placed on the patient. Reported loss events entailed physical or emotional separations from significant persons in patients' lives; changes in expectations often derived from situations in which patients were asked to take on increased responsibilities in their occupations. Further exploration suggested that these events were linked to frightening experiences in childhood and that the patients viewed them as threats to important attachment figures. Seven of the nine patients had difficulty acknowledging their angry feelings. Sexual conflicts were not prominent in panic onset in this study; when present, they appeared to be secondary to fears regarding attachment and anger. Patients perceived their parents as controlling, frightening, temperamental, critical, and demanding. Every patient described significant problems in relationships with other persons, and seven of the nine reported occupation-related difficulties.

In a further review of the interviews, Shear et al. (1993) found that patients revealed themes of early life anxiety and shyness, unsupportive parental relationships, and a chronic sense of feeling trapped and troubled by frustration and resentment. Most patients described feelings of inadequacy or self-reproach. Aggression was prominent and uncomfortable; patients often attempted to manage it with efforts to undo complaints or turn negative attributes into positive qualities.

In the formulation described by Busch et al. (1991) and Shear et al. (1993), one of two scenarios may apply to patients at risk for panic disorder. An individual may have a neurophysiological vulnerability to panic—manifested in early life as behavioral inhibition to the unfamiliar, as defined by Kagan et al. (1990) and Rosenbaum et al. (1988). Alternatively, an otherwise unremarkable individual may experience a series of traumatic developmental events.

Patients with behavioral inhibition are frightened by unfamiliarities in the environment and rely on parents to provide a sense of safety; because parents cannot always provide this comfort, these patients develop a sense of fearful dependence on their parents. These patients experience fear of the unfamiliar as narcissistic injuries and blame their inadequacies on their parents, whom they view as unreliable. In individuals with an unremarkable disposition, a parent's actual rejecting or controlling behavior can produce a state of fearful dependence in the child.

In either scenario, the child becomes angry at the parent's rejecting or frightening behavior. As a result, the child becomes fearful of loss and frightened that his or her angry fantasies will destroy the parent on whom he or she depends. In this vicious cycle, rage threatens the all-important tie to the parent and increases the child's fearful dependence. This process leads to further frustration and rage at the parent, whom the child views as the source of his or her inadequacies.

Immaturity or failure of the ego's signal anxiety function leads to the uncontrollable onset of panic levels of anxiety. The signal anxiety function is an intrapsychic mechanism, posited by Freud (1926/1950), that generates smaller doses of anxiety to alert the ego to the presence of psychologically meaningful dangers and act as a stimulus to mobilize defenses; this process prevents the experience of overwhelming anxiety. This cycle is repeated in adulthood, when threats to attachment trigger regression.

This formulation is corroborated by two sources: patients' retrospective views of their interactions and prospective direct systematic research. As such, although speculative, it provides a working model that has potential power to explain the meaning of patients' habitual actions and symptoms.

Shear et al. (1993) also described variations in patients' dependence conflicts. Some vulnerable individuals, for example, are "separation sensitive" or overly reliant on others. Others appear to be "suffocation sensitive" (Klein 1993). Suffocation-sensitive persons are uncomfortable about their unconscious dependence needs, which they feel are overwhelming; consequently, they feel engulfed or controlled by others. In either case, however, defenses remain immature and are easily overwhelmed. Patients tend to experience anger and guilt connected with their preoccupying fantasies of being abandoned or trapped by the people on whom they desperately depend. Negative affects are uncomfortable and often avoided. This emotional backdrop fosters patients' focus on somatic, rather than psychic, discomfort.

Milrod (1995) posited that in some patients, in addition to conflicts surrounding attachment and anger, panic episodes have a frightening and arousing inherent excitement—often closely tied to sadomasochistic sexual conflicts and characterological traits. We discuss this issue in more depth in Chapter 5.

The following case is an example of a psychological history of panic onset. We found this pattern to be typical of these patients.

Case Example

Ms. A—a 31-year-old, single, white health care provider—described the onset of panic attacks with fears of dying from a heart attack a few days after observing the sudden death of a patient. Ms. A noted gruesome particulars of the death, although she had not experienced significant anxiety previously when she had seen patients die. She reported feeling particularly close to this patient; a closer inquiry, however, revealed that she knew little about the patient's life. Ms. A found the "unfairness" of the patient's death particularly upsetting: the patient was young, recovering, and planning for discharge when she died. Ms. A thought, "God, you can't do this to her." Ms. A subsequently developed the fear that she or someone she knew could die suddenly.

In reviewing her history of anxiety, Ms. A denied that she was "an anxious person," although people who knew her felt she was anxious. She proceeded to reveal recurrent, intense fears about her health over many years, although these fears had not previously manifested in the form of panic attacks. In addition, Ms. A routinely experienced anxiety in traffic jams or crowded department stores. She also noted that she was shy when young and frightened of other children.

In response to inquiry into other areas of her life, Ms. A revealed multiple other stresses that preoccupied her at the time of panic onset. For example, she felt she was unfairly treated at her job; she felt she was paid less and worked longer hours than colleagues at similar jobs in other hospitals. Ms. A also was in a problematic relationship with her boyfriend. She described him as "cold and callous," and she felt that he was not responding to her efforts in the relationship: "I gave 150% and he gave 10%."

When asked about her home life growing up, Ms. A described a volatile, terrifying father. Her father yelled at her mother, her siblings, and her. She was disturbed by his behavior and determined that she would never marry a man like him. Ms. A's mother was a "nervous person" who was frightened about her children's health and safety and felt a need to keep things hidden from Ms. A's father. Ms. A frequently exclaimed to her mother, "Ma, you're worrying yourself to death." The following exchange illustrates some aspects of the patient's anxiety:

Therapist: Were your mother's worries similar to the ones you had when you were panicking?

Patient: I think I get it from my mother. I became worried that others would be hurt. My sister and I would go out without my father's knowledge. If she were late in meeting me, I'd think, "Oh my God, she's dead. They're going to kill me."

Therapist: There's a lot of death and killing in your language.

Patient: Yes, I don't know where that comes from.

Ms. A reported that she frequently felt deprived as a child. When she did not get what she demanded, she cried, sulked, and "became anxious." She complained, "I got the short end of the stick from a very young age"—particularly compared with her younger sister, who was more assertive and popular. Ms. A said she was upset when her sister received things from their parents before she did, despite the fact that Ms. A was older.

Ms. A had tremendous difficulty discussing her angry feelings. She minimized her anger and frequently followed an angry comment with a disclaimer. For instance, she noted that she often held grudges against people—but then remarked that she was not "vindictive." In response to questions about her "get even" fantasies, Ms. A reluctantly revealed thoughts of blowing up her former boyfriend's car:

Patient: But I would never hope that he died. I'm not like that.

Therapist: Is there a difference between the kinds of things you imagine happening to someone you're enraged with, like this ex-boyfriend, and the kinds of things you imagine happening to you when you're having your worst panic, or are they similar kinds of things?

Patient: I'd say they're similar.

Ms. A subsequently said that she had always wanted to help people. "I've always been the helping kind," she commented.

At the end of the interview, Ms. A appeared calmer and seemed more curious about her panic symptoms. "There's a lot you keep inside of you, and panic gets it out," she said. "Maybe it is the way I was brought up. I thought it was just that one incident."

This case illustrates typical findings among patients experiencing panic that we interviewed in this study. The panic occurred subsequent to a specific incident—in this case, the death of a patient—and in the context of multiple stresses in the patient's work and relationships. The precipitating event in this case, as in others, also had important meanings for the patient that were connected to her own history, particularly with regard to developmental and characterological themes and reactions to "unfairness." Ms. A, for example, experienced her patient's untimely death, the conditions of her job (in which she was "underpaid and overworked"), and her relationship with her boyfriend—in which she "gave 150% and he gave 10%"—as unfair. When Ms. A was growing up, she felt deprived, particularly with regard to her younger sister—whom she saw as unfairly getting many things that she did not have. Ms. A noted that she felt anxious when she became angry about what she perceived as mistreatment by her parents. (There was not enough time in the initial interview to explore the possible psychological links between the woman who died and the patient's sister.)

Ms. A's description of her family background was typical of the circumstances in panic patients' families. This environment included a temperamental and frightening father, of whom everyone—including the patient—was terrified, as well as an anxious mother. Thus, Ms. A grew up in an atmosphere in which anxiety was chronic and intense and anger was poorly controlled. She also described longstanding anxieties about her health and being in crowded situations.

Ms. A was wrestling with intense angry feelings in the interview. Initially reluctant to describe her fantasies of revenge, she later maintained that she was "not that kind of person" and in fact was "the helping kind." (We discuss further such efforts to manage anger via undoing and reaction formation in Chapter 6.) Clearly, Ms. A was intensely angry at people she felt were treating her unfairly at the time, including her boyfriend and the hospital where she worked. Given her discomfort about her anger, the experience of that anger probably contributed to the onset of her panic. The interviewer elicited from Ms. A the connection between her rage-filled fantasies and the damage that she expected to occur to her when she was panicking. The patient's rage and anxiety at her father's frightening and aggressive behavior would be a likely source of further elaboration about important aspects of her panic (although it could not be explored in the initial interview).

Like many other patients, Ms. A became increasingly interested about the developmental and psychological contributions to the onset of her panic. In this study, we found that patients' understanding that there were specific psychological sources to the onset of their panic appeared to help relieve their anxiety. In our view, the ability to describe and explore intense affective states of rage and loss associated with panic onset helped to reduce patients' anxiety about these highly conflicted feelings.

Substantial evidence suggests that psychological factors have a central role in the genesis and onset of panic disorder, as well as the frequency of relapse after treatment termination. In the following chapters, we present a series of techniques and illustrations of psychodynamic treatment of patients with panic disorder. Although we offer general principles for this type of therapy, the approaches that clinicians use will vary depending on their patients' individual life histories, conflicts, and life situations.

Chapter 3

Overview of Treatment

In this manual, we provide detailed descriptions of methods of exploratory psychotherapy for patients with panic disorder. In panic-focused psychodynamic psychotherapy (PFPP), the therapist maintains a sustained focus on the symptoms of panic attacks and accompanying agoraphobia. Early in the treatment, the therapist actively pursues the patient's experiences as they relate to panic onset. We describe specific techniques and common problems that can interfere with this treatment. We also include a discussion of techniques that may be necessary with patients who externalize their problems, as well as a description of common countertransference difficulties.

Clinicians can use PFPP as a brief psychotherapy, aimed at rapid elimination of panic symptoms, or as a longer-term treatment designed to address vulnerability to panic relapse and functional impairment. We outline aspects of treatment of both lengths.

Research studies typically involve short-term (approximately 3-month) treatment of patients, with resolution of panic attacks as the primary goal. Although a brief treatment provides some insight into the underlying origin of symptoms, therapists can explore vulnerability to panic only in a limited way in this time frame. In clinical practice, therapists and patients often recognize that continued treatment is required to address the chronic, debilitating characterological difficulties and conflicts that lead to panic onset—and necessarily affect other areas of the patient's life. Longer-term treatment can uncover significant unconscious dynamisms that are responsible for the predisposition to symptom formation. Psychotherapy can help the patient to understand these dynamisms, which then may be subject to modification.

The current health care climate often dictates brief treatment. In our experience, however, lengthier psychotherapeutic treatment often brings patients significantly greater benefit with fewer exacerbations of acute panic and reduced need for further medical and psychiatric interventions. Therefore, although PFPP is designed to be used in a brief form (approximately 3 months) for relief of acute panic symptoms, it may be expanded to be a longer-term treatment (9–12 months) aimed at vulnerability to panic relapse. Furthermore, patients with panic disorder who have severe personality disorders may require treatment for more than 12 months to address panic vulnerability (see Chapter 9).

We intend that this manual will be used by qualified professionals who are in the midst of training or have completed clinical training in Accreditation Council of Graduate Medical Education–approved psychiatric residency training programs, American Psychological Association–approved psychology training programs, or approved social work training programs. Adequate supervision by qualified, psychodynamically trained supervisors must be available for optimal use of PFPP—whether in clinical practice or in research.

Summary of Treatment

In the first phase of treatment, interventions are aimed at exploring and relieving panic attacks (see Table 3–1). The therapist focuses on the circumstances preceding panic onset, the patient's thoughts and feelings during panic attacks, and the meanings of panic symptoms. As this exploration proceeds, the therapist can formulate psychologically meaningful issues involved in the genesis of the patient's panic episodes; these issues may include conflicts about separation, anger, and sexuality (as described earlier).

Our clinical experience—as well as a review of cases in the literature—suggests that this approach usually provides relief of panic symptoms in approximately 12–20 weeks of exploratory psychotherapy (Milrod and Shear 1991a, 1991b). Agoraphobic symptoms (if present) sometimes resolve more slowly, although agoraphobia often resolves with panic attacks. This outcome is comparable with results reported with cognitive-behavioral and psychopharmacological treatments.

In the second phase of treatment, the therapist explores in greater depth the mental configurations that elicit the patient's panic

Table 3–1. Panic-focused psychodynamic psychotherapy (The number of sessions allotted to different phases of treatment will vary from patient to patient.)

Phase I: Treatment of acute panic. To lessen panic symptoms, we believe that it is necessary to uncover the unconscious meaning of these symptoms. The following strategy is used:

- A. Initial evaluation and early treatment
  1. Exploration of circumstances and feelings surrounding panic onset
  2. Exploration of personal meanings of panic symptoms
  3. Exploration of feelings and content of panic episodes
- B. Psychodynamic conflicts in panic disorder
  1. Separation and independence
  2. Anger recognition, management, and coping with expression
  3. Sexual excitement and its perceived dangers
- C. Expected responses to Phase I of treatment
  1. Panic symptom relief
  2. Reduction in agoraphobic symptoms

Phase II: Treatment of panic vulnerability. To lessen vulnerability to panic, we hypothesize that core dynamisms must be understood and altered. To do this, these dynamisms must be identified with the patient in the course of the psychotherapy, often through their emergence in the transference. The following strategy is used:

- A. Addressing conflicts in the transference
- B. Working through
- C. Expected responses to Phase II of treatment
  1. Improvement in relationships
  2. Less conflicted experience of separation, anger, sexuality
  3. Reduction in vulnerability to panic recurrence

Phase III: Termination. To address panic patients' severe difficulties with separation and independence, we hypothesize that the experience of termination in this time-limited psychotherapy will permit the patient to re-experience these conflicts directly with the therapist so that underlying fantasies can begin to be

(Table 3–1 continues)

Table 3–1. Panic-focused psychodynamic psychotherapy *(continued)*

articulated, understood, and rendered less frightening. Patient reaction to termination must be addressed for a minimum of the final third of the treatment.

A. Re-experiencing of central separation and anger themes in the transference as termination approaches
B. Expected responses to Phase II of treatment
    1. Possible temporary recrudescence of symtoms as these feelings are experienced in therapy
    2. New ability to manage separations and independence

symptoms and the characterological underpinnings to these symptoms. As the patient's unconscious conflicts emerge in therapy, the therapist and the patient actively seek to uncover dynamic connections with emotional configurations that occur during panic episodes. During this phase, intensification of the transference allows for increasing work on patterns in relationships, as they emerge in the relationship with the therapist. The goal of this phase of psychotherapy is to reduce the patient's vulnerability to panic relapse through further conscious delineation of the interpersonal emotional script with which patients conduct their lives. We hypothesize that most dynamics related to panic vulnerability can be addressed successfully in a 9-month to 1-year period.

These phases of therapy may be divided, to some extent, into earlier and later periods of treatment. Furthermore, the focus may vary significantly for different patients. For example, transference may emerge as a prominent focus quite early in the treatment of some patients.

Although we do not describe longer-term psychodynamic psychotherapeutic treatment in this manual, a few case vignettes in the text involve patients who were treated initially with PFPP who continued to pursue longer-term psychotherapy. Therapists can conduct such longer-term treatment using the same principles as those described here. Such longer-term psychotherapy no longer focuses on panic symptoms, as initial treatment did; instead, it includes other aspects of the patient's life. The therapist further investigates patients' characterological disturbances and conflicts. The goal of this type of treatment is to help patients address more widespread characterological disturbances as they affect interpersonal relationships and professional life.

Chapter 4

Initial Evaluation and Early Sessions

Initial Evaluation

The initial evaluation of a patient with panic disorder includes an assessment of panic attacks and associated anxiety symptoms. The therapist also must evaluate the patient's ability to benefit from psychodynamic psychotherapy. The psychodynamically oriented clinician explores the patient's character, life history, level of functioning, and perception of significant relationships. A patient's ability to express himself or herself in words is an important aspect of his or her ability to benefit from the process of psychodynamic psychotherapy. In the evaluation, the therapist conducts a semi-structured interview, paying particular attention to topics that make the patient uncomfortable or defensive.

The following guidelines cover areas that we have found important in panic assessment. Clinicians need not adhere rigidly to these guidelines, however.

1) Assessment of panic attacks
    a) DSM-IV (American Psychiatric Association 1994) symptoms
    b) Situations preceding panic onset: circumstances, feelings, stressors (losses, changes in location, alteration in level of responsibilities, relationships with significant others)
    c) Prior panic episodes with symptoms, thoughts, feelings, circumstances of onset
2) Developmental history
    a) Perception of parents and family life, focusing on how the family managed anger, anxiety, and other emotional topics; history of early losses and separations

   b) Childhood anxiety symptoms: school phobias, shyness, childhood fears and worries
   c) Adolescence: dependence/independence conflicts, relationships, struggles concerning control, autonomy, anxiety management; how anger, separation, and sexuality were handled
   d) Adult relationships: types and quality of relationships that patients conduct with significant others, including nature of conflicts, level of responsibility with which the patient is comfortable, and assertiveness versus passivity in most major relationships
3) Assessment of the patient's capacity to make use of psychotherapy, including the patient's ability to think psychologically, describe relations to others, make dynamic connections, put feelings into words, and maintain curiosity about his or her motivation and role in his or her difficulties.

The patient's motivation to work in psychotherapy and take the process seriously is important (Malan 1979). Motivation typically is high for panic patients when they begin a new treatment; when patients experience a high degree of distress, they are quite ready to work in therapy. The therapist should note dynamic themes that emerge during the evaluation process to assess the patient's ability to make connections regarding the psychological meanings of panic.

Case Example

Mr. B sought treatment for his crippling panic disorder only when the severity of his panic attacks, agoraphobia, and obsessional ruminations had become so compelling that he had to drop out of college. At the time of his first therapy session, he was preoccupied with the fantasy that he had acquired AIDS during a social encounter with a homosexual male friend, during which they had watched pornographic movies together. Although he was aware as he entered the office that the concern about AIDS probably was unreasonable, he was initially unable to expand further about the reasons for his anxiety.

Therapist: From what you've described just now in your history, it sounds like you're frequently this anxious, but that your specific concerns change.

Patient: Well, that's true. But now, I think that the other things I've worried about in the past were silly compared to this. [*Pause.*] You know what, though? I always think that, no matter what I'm worried about.

Therapist: It sounds like you think there's a pattern to the process of your anxious concerns.

Patient: If you had said that to me yesterday, I wouldn't have agreed. But now that you say that, I think I'm starting to think that it's true. Bottom line, I always think I'm going nuts.

Therapist: Do you have any idea why you tend to think these things?

Patient: No. Well, yes, actually. I think my parents are crazy and that they've messed me up somehow.

Therapist: That sounds like quite a disturbing fantasy.

Patient: Well, I guess it is. How'd I get like that?

In this exchange, the patient indicated that he had the capacity to think about his feelings in a more objective, detached way and that he could connect past emotions with his current situation. Mr. B demonstrated his curiosity to understand why he had these disturbing fantasies. Within this brief interchange, he was able to connect his symptoms with fantasies that he had about himself and his family, and he followed the therapist's exploratory leads by pursuing underlying thoughts. Although a therapist generally cannot conclusively determine the patient's capacity to make use of psychodynamic treatment within the first encounter, the characteristics demonstrated by this patient, including curiosity, the ability to step back and look at his feelings, and his interest in the therapist's ideas, are important early indicators about him.

In contrast to cognitive-behavioral treatments, psychodynamic treatment of panic does not focus on psychoeducation. Nevertheless, some cognitive-behavioral and psychoeducational techniques often are explicit in this treatment. For example, during the evaluation the clinician should make an educational statement about the diagnosis and neurophysiological underpinnings of the disorder. The therapist also should discuss treatment options with the patient; if the therapist considers psychodynamic psychotherapy to be appropriate—based on factors outlined earlier—the therapist should encourage the patient to pursue this treatment. At the end of the evaluation, the clinician may offer the patient a psychodynamic life narrative formulation (Viederman and Perry 1980), with a dynamic description of the meaning of panic.

The therapist should be calm, assured, and empathic with the patient. In offering information to the patient, the therapist should state clearly what the problem is and how treatment will address it. The therapist should be active in educating the patient about how psychotherapy works: for example, the therapist should point out that dreams, free associations, and fantasies may be important mental constellations that can be used to explore unconscious fantasies. We recommend treatment at least twice weekly; this frequency allows the patient to achieve a relationship of sufficient intensity with the therapist for transference interventions to carry convincing emotional weight.

Relationship With the Therapist

A panic patient may have special problems in developing a therapeutic alliance. For many patients with panic disorder, the establishment of an alliance with the therapist will be the most frightening—as well as the most important—part of treatment. This relationship is established over time; the therapist's openness and willingness to discuss the patient's symptoms and concerns will foster such an alliance. The therapist should take seriously the patient's questions about how the treatment works and carefully explain the process. This attitude is important throughout the treatment, although patient confusion about the treatment process becomes increasingly influenced by transferential fantasies as therapy progresses. The therapist should observe the evolution of transference against the backdrop of this helpful, professional, yet friendly relationship.

Patients with panic disorder are intensely anxious; they often require a significant amount of reassurance that their problems can be treated effectively. Therapists should not feel inhibited about providing this reassurance: They should tell patients that panic symptoms typically respond well to treatment. Although reassurance and psychoeducation are essential tools in all treatments, psychodynamic psychotherapy uses these techniques to calm patients enough for the therapist to explore the underlying meaning of symptoms.

Engaging the Patient

Some patients readily engage in the psychotherapeutic process in an effort to understand the psychological origins of their panic attacks. Others, however, because of character style or a failure to see the relevance of psychological issues to their panic attacks, show little interest. Often, the therapist can engage the patient's interest and curiosity by demonstrating how panic symptoms may be related to the patient's current and past mode of behavior. The therapist can connect the patient's panic with emotional concerns that the patient has had throughout his or her life.

Case Example

During the course of her initial evaluation, Ms. C, a 28-year-old woman, said that she failed to see the relevance that her relationship with her mother had in connection with her panic attacks. This attitude was striking because she described her mother as controlling and suffocating, and she experienced the sensation of suffocation during her panic attacks. Ms. C lived alone with her mother and constantly struggled with her. The therapist approached this topic with a careful exploration of the precise experience that Ms. C had during panic episodes; Ms. C mentioned that she would begin to scratch her skin.

Therapist: Can you tell me something about that experience?

Patient: Yes, I feel very upset at that point. But I'm not sure why I do it.

Therapist: Have you experienced this feeling or behavior at any other point?

Patient: Well, yes: when I'm upset at someone and in a fight. But I'm not panicking then. I have it when I'm fighting with my mother.

Therapist: What do you think it means for you then?

Patient: Well, it gets her to be quiet. It's one of the only ways to get her to stop attacking me. Yes, that's quite interesting that it's the same as in my panic attacks. In some ways, I experience some of the same things when I'm fighting with my mother that I feel when I'm panicking, although I'm more angry than anxious. After the fight, my mother stops talking to me, and I begin to feel like a terrible person. That's when the panic feelings start.

This realization was an important stage in Ms. C's treatment. It marked a new awareness of the connection between the subjective experience of suffocation, her rage with her mother, and how both were related to her emotional state during her panic attacks.

The capacity to be psychologically minded is an important part of psychodynamic psychotherapeutic work. The therapist must evaluate this capacity in the patient by providing useful examples of psychological factors that emerge in the patient's panic experience, as illustrated earlier. If the patient can make use of this material, he or she will likely elaborate on the formulations presented by the therapist, adding details and altering the formulation to apply to his or her situation more exactly.

Humiliation Concerning Symptoms

Patients with panic disorder often experience significant feelings of humiliation about their panic symptoms. These feelings constitute a common source of difficulty in engaging panic patients in treatment. Patients with these symptoms commonly are invested in thinking of themselves as "strong" and have high expectations of themselves about having control over their feelings. This embarrassment reflects the fact that panic attacks frequently make people feel incapacitated, immature, and weak. This emotional configuration can be a barrier to engaging in treatment because patients often feel too embarrassed to acknowledge the extent of their symptoms to anyone, including themselves or their therapist.

Therapists must be aware of the extent to which patients feel the need to deny their symptoms. Gradually, opportunities arise in therapy that enable patients to acknowledge how much the anxiety symptoms they have been trying to avoid are curtailing their lives.

Case Example

Mr. D, a 30-year-old man, had always seen himself as a "strong person." He felt that he needed to be strong and that he and others would view any sign of weakness as humiliating. Mr. D felt that his parents expected him never to demonstrate weakness. He described his father—whom he took a model for his behavior—as "never getting upset or depressed." Mr. D's panic attacks developed in the context of a series of stressors, including his marriage and a promotion at work that entailed greater responsibilities. He was frightened that he would be unable to perform at his new job and would be fired. As his anxiety mounted, he became increasingly worried that he would be rejected or abandoned by his wife because he needed her help. This conflict added to his feelings of abandonment and panic because he felt more alone and in danger of losing everything.

Therapist: How did your wife respond to your telling her about your anxiety?

Patient: Oh, really well. She was very supportive. But I had the sense that she would get sick of it, especially as I went on and on.

Therapist: You really don't feel she can handle your anxiety.

Patient: [*Tearful*] No. Deep down, I don't feel she can. I just feel that she will see me as weak and lose interest.

Therapist: You seem to feel that when you need help, there is no way to express it without risking being abandoned by others.

Patient: Yes, I think that's true. And I know that she is responsive to me. But, I don't know. I've always felt I needed to be strong. Maybe I can try to let that go a little.

Mr. D's panic attacks resolved after 2 weeks of therapy. He remained in weekly psychotherapy for 6 months to address issues related to his vulnerability to panic.

Case Example

Ms. E, a 21-year-old student, came to psychotherapy for a variety of pressing anxiety symptoms, including panic attacks and an embarrassing fear of being alone or driving a car. A tough-talking late teenager, she prided herself on always being rational, unlike her girlfriends or her mother. Ms. E admitted that her anxiety symptoms were highly embarrassing to her and that, in fact, they were the part of herself that she most disliked. Nevertheless, she had extreme difficulty talking about her scary thoughts and fantasies in therapy. The therapist found herself asking about Ms. E's symptoms often, while Ms. E smiled pleasantly and minimized their impact.

Gathering information about the fantasies underlying Ms. E's anxiety remained difficult for quite some time; she said that she could not remember thoughts that were connected in any way with the symptoms. She remembered no dreams from any point in her life. Ms. E said that she was in less distress because she had started her therapy, but the reasons for this improvement remained obscure. "I just need to keep coming," she said; "I don't know why." Her panic attacks had resolved 2 weeks after she began psychotherapy.

The following month, she planned to move to another city for a summer job; she arranged to live with her best friend. Weeks in therapy were taken up with the details of her summer apartment and work. The therapist said that Ms. E seemed to believe that the summer would liberate her from many of her concerns, including her school work as well as her anxiety symptoms, which she continued to describe as having been in the past. Ms. E agreed merrily.

One week after leaving for the other city (2 months after her initial presentation), Ms. E called her therapist, saying that she would be in town the next week and would like to see her. When she came to the office, Ms. E said that things had "kind of gone wrong in [the other city]" and that she had been shocked by how upset and frightened she had been there. She had changed her mind, given up her summer plans, and decided she would continue to live at home with her parents for the summer. She sheepishly said that she would resume therapy for the summer.

Patient: It's really not that big a deal, though; I just like it here.

Therapist: Well, it is rather a surprise. I know how much you were looking forward to your summer plans.

Patient: Yeah, I was, but I figured out that I just didn't want to be there. And it's no problem with Marcy; she's not mad. I helped her to find another roommate. So it's fine.

Therapist: I can tell that you don't want this summer to be a big deal, but I really think it's important for us to look at exactly what happened in [the other city]. It seems familiar because we've just been talking about how, so often, you really try to hide the extent of your worries even from yourself.

Patient: Yeah, it is what we've been saying. [*Laughs with bravado*]

Therapist: Well, I think that the sudden change of plans gives us the opportunity here to explore what happens for you when you get really scared. I know that this whole experience must make you feel very embarrassed, like you're a baby, right at a time when you've been trying to be more independent from your parents. I do think, though, that if we don't explore it better than we've done up to now it will probably happen again, and I know you really don't want that.

Patient: I know. I just have to move out of my parents' house soon. This can't keep happening!

After this point, Ms. E finally became more engaged and curious about her own thoughts, which were so frightening to her; only then could she more effectively use her therapy in an exploratory manner. This case is particularly illustrative: the patient's panic attacks disappeared almost immediately when she began psychotherapy, although she had not gained any substantive understanding about them. Thus, the "cure" was at risk of backfiring, given the extent of the patient's intolerance of the acknowledgment of her symptoms and her unwillingness to confront the role played by separation fears in her panic onset. The reemergence of symptoms when she interrupted her therapy, even briefly, was predictable.

Early Sessions

Panic-focused psychodynamic psychotherapy initially targets the psychological meanings surrounding panic disorder and its onset.

Most commonly, patients begin early sessions with descriptions of panic symptoms because these symptoms often are compelling. A variety of probes are useful in this situation:

- What occurs to you about the panic as you talk about it now?
- What do you think you could have been worried about?
- What comes to mind about specific points?

If patients do not begin by describing their panic attacks, the therapist eventually should pursue the symptoms and attempt to relate that information to panic states. Primary areas of focus in treatment include feelings and circumstances surrounding panic onset, the meanings of individual panic symptoms, and feelings and thoughts accompanying panic episodes.

In the course of psychotherapy, patterns emerge regarding particular stresses and thoughts and feelings that precede panic, which the therapist must communicate to the patient. The therapist may make brief connections—for example, "So, at the time of your first symptoms you were dining with a friend at a restaurant that called up specific memories," or "At the time of your first attack, you were alone in your room reading something that stirred up a specific disturbing thought."

Stressors Preceding Panic Onset

Panic patients often describe their symptoms as having come "out of the blue," with no clear origin. Many researchers, backed by the DSM description of panic disorder, appear to have accepted these statements as representing the actual nature of the illness. Life event studies of clinical interviews (discussed in Chapter 2), however, suggest that meaningful life events typically precede panic onset. In our experience, a patient's belief that the illness came "out of the blue" represents a defense against the intense emotions that the precipitating events have engendered. The therapist must explore with the patient life events that led to panic onset and their emotional significance.

Case Example

Ms. F, a 16-year-old mother of a 1-year-old, presented to a hospital emergency department complaining of the sudden onset of "confusional events" during the preceding 3 weeks. The initial evaluation, which included a neurological workup because of Ms. F's choice of focus in describing her symptoms, revealed that she was having panic attacks for the first time in her life. The attacks included prominent feelings of loss of balance and tachycardia, as well as a sense of impending doom. Initially, Ms. F could think of nothing different in her emotional life that could have been responsible for these changes.

Therapist: So, you really can't think of any way in which your life is different or has changed since you started having the panic attacks?

Patient: No. There's nothing. I just sit at home with my daughter. I have a boring life.

Therapist: What are your plans?

Patient: Well, actually, I've been thinking of joining the army lately. I've gotten all the material. I just received it in the mail last month. It looks great; they'll pay for me to go to college and graduate school. It's really going to be the only way I can afford to do what I want.

Therapist: What'll happen to the baby?

Patient: I can leave her with my grandmother during the week and see her on the weekends. It's not ideal, but of course, it was ridiculous for me not to get an abortion given my age.

Therapist: What does your husband think of your plans?

Patient: Oh, he's hysterical, actually. He thinks he'll lose me. He wants me to stay home. I'm sure that's why he wanted to get me pregnant in the first place, come to think of it. But this is my *life*! I have to go. It will break my heart not to be around the baby, but in the end it's for her good.

Therapist: And your grandmother?

Patient: [*Laughing*] She's pretty upset too. They love me. They don't want me to go away. I've never been away at all, ever.

Therapist: When was all of this to take place?

Patient: Well, before I got sick, I was in the middle of applying. It was supposed to be for next month. I've had to put it off now.

Therapist: With all of this in the air, I'm particularly struck by your saying that nothing's different in your life.

Patient: [*Laughing*] So, you really think this is connected?

Therapist: Yes.

Patient: Well, I hate to admit it, but I guess I've been a little scared lately. Things were suddenly going so fast. The idea of not seeing the baby almost kills me.

The Psychological Meaning of Symptoms

DSM-IV describes a list of symptoms that, taken together, define the syndrome of panic disorder. Patients who meet the criteria for panic disorder vary, however, with regard to their symptomatic profile, and panic thoughts that accompany the attacks vary considerably in their specific content, despite their universal theme of catastrophe. Minor individual variations in the syndrome often carry specific psychological meanings for patients. The therapist should explore each symptom in depth with regard to its origins and psychological meanings.

Case Example

Ms. G experienced "typical" panic symptoms of shortness of breath and palpitations. She feared that she would suddenly die. Both of her parents had died at relatively young ages; her father died in a car accident, and her mother died of cancer. Ms. G's profession, which entailed work with terminally ill patients, aggravated her sense of a lack of safety about her body with the feeling that it was prone to sudden deterioration.

Patient: Maybe having death so near at hand gets me more frightened. The scariest feeling is the shortness of breath. As soon as I experience that, I begin to panic.

Therapist: What does this experience bring to mind?

Patient: Well, when my mother was dying from cancer, she became very short of breath. It was terrible seeing her that way because it was at that point she realized that she was going to die. She became very tearful. I couldn't bear it.

Therapist: Had you ever seen her like that before?

Patient: No. Not quite like that. But after my father died she cried frequently. She was very helpless, and I had to take over things around the house. That was a terrible time for my siblings and me. It's interesting because I also feel helpless when I panic. I wonder if my shortness of breath is so scary because of what happened to my mother.

Ms. G's panic attacks occurred after she had recollections of her mother, triggered by cleaning out her parents' home so she could sell it. This experience, combined with other losses at that time, led to memories of the painful experiences of losing her mother—at first emotionally, when her father died, and later through death. In fantasy, Ms. G had re-created these moments repeatedly during her panic attacks.

Case Example

Ms. H said that one of her greatest fears during her panic attacks was that she would choke and suffocate while drinking. She revealed that when she was angry at other people, she often experienced the sense that she was physically suffocating. In therapy, she recalled intense, angry struggles at the dinner table during her childhood about whether she was eating and drinking enough.

Patient: I remember I wouldn't drink or eat my food. My father would get very angry and scream at me to drink. I felt forced to do it, like I might choke. I was really mad and crying.

Therapist: Did it feel anything like the experience of choking in panic attacks?

Patient: Yes, I guess it did, but I don't think I was panicking then. My father and I were always fighting over the years, and I often had that feeling.

These experiences became part of a combative, exciting, sadomasochistic relationship with her father, which contributed to her anxiety. At the beginning of treatment, Ms. H had discussed a hierarchy of frightening situations; choking while drinking was at the top of the list. Ms. H experienced her panic attacks, along with feelings of suffocation, after experiences in which there were angry, exciting conflicts with her boyfriend.

Feelings During Panic

Although current definitions of panic disorder emphasize feelings of intense anxiety, our clinical data suggest that patients often experience a wide array of feelings during panic episodes. Several investigators (Fava et al. 1990; George et al. 1989; McGrath et al. 1985) have described so-called anger attacks as a variant of panic disorder. In our experience, constellations of inhibited angry feelings frequently are a conscious and unconscious accompaniment to panic. Moreover, we have found that panic symptoms often carry other emotional valences. For example, they can symbolize an ambivalent longing for an absent object, among other things. A thorough dynamic workup of panic disorder must include an exploration of these topics.

Another common feeling during panic attacks is humiliation about perceived loss of control. Patients often experience a sense of confusion during these episodes. The therapist should try to elicit the feelings that occur during panic attacks because these feelings form the emotional web that brings about the symptoms.

Case Example

Mr. I, a 38-year-old man, worried that he would leave his lover, even though he didn't want to, because of his chronic feelings of jealousy. This feeling resembled his experiences in past love relationships. One evening, Mr. I's lover did not seem to be as responsive as usual. Mr. I feared that his lover would suddenly end the relationship. He described a frightening feeling of potential loss. In this context, he had a panic attack.

Therapist: Tell me more about what frightened you in the situation.

Patient: Well, I was very worried about how frightened I was. I felt crazy, and I was very embarrassed about it. I worried he would find out how crazy I was.

Therapist: And then what did you think would happen?

Patient: Well, then he would reject me for how crazy I was, if he wasn't going to do it anyway. But rationally, I know there was really no problem at all. He wasn't about to end the relationship. Then later I was worried that I had offended him.

Therapist: In what way?

Patient: I asked him: Why are you behaving this way? I worried that offended him.

Therapist: You said it an angry way?

Patient: Yes, I guess I was angry at him. I don't like to admit that. I had a lot of different feelings. It was very confusing.

As the therapist explored Mr. I's feelings further, the patient reported an increasingly complex array of emotions during his panic episode. Each feeling contributed to the experience of the panic state. The exploration in psychotherapy helped to reveal multiple roots of the patient's intense fears of loss and doom.

This example demonstrates the complexity of possible transformations of anger. Mr. I had frequent thoughts of leaving his lover because he was jealous, yet he interpreted his lover's unresponsiveness as anger at him, which led him to fear that he would be abandoned. This common mechanism of projection, which serves to undo the passivity of dependent feelings, also functioned as a punishment for conflicted fantasies of straying or for angry feelings.

Early Treatment

The following case illustrates aspects of the first several sessions in the psychodynamic treatment of a panic patient:

Case Example

Ms. G (a patient mentioned earlier) presented with panic attacks for which she had a full medical work-up. The medical examination was negative, but she still was not certain that she was medically safe. At first, the therapist reassured her about the nature of her illness.

Therapist: Your symptoms are consistent with what we call panic disorder, which is a treatable psychiatric illness. The symptoms that you describe—shortness of breath and palpitations—are part of this disorder, rather than signs of a medical disease.

Patient: Well, that's very reassuring to know. It seemed as if I must have been having a heart attack.

This educational step had a calming effect on the patient, and the therapist proceeded with exploring the situation at the time of panic onset. Ms. G said that she did not understand why she had the onset of panic because there were no particularly difficult problems in her life at that time. In response to the therapist's questions, however, she revealed that she had been cleaning out her parents' house to sell it, but had been "too busy" to let it bother her. She also reported that she had realized that a 15-year relationship with her boyfriend was "not going to go anywhere" but that this was no "boo-hoo." She initially denied having any problems at her job, although she later said that she dealt with critically ill patients in her work (an "emotional drain") and was on the verge of changing jobs.

Therapist: What was it like closing up your parents' home?

Patient: Well, it was very busy. We didn't have time to think of anything.

Therapist: When was your first panic attack?

Patient: The day after we closed the house.

Therapist: Did cleaning up the house bring up memories of your parents' death?

Patient: Oh yes. We all talked about it. My father died suddenly when I was age 18. It was very hard on my mother, having to care for all of us. I couldn't stand seeing her like that. Later, I became very angry with my father; he left us with a lot of debts. [*Begins to cry*] Then my mother died of cancer when she was only 55. It was terrible to see her when she realized she was going to die. It was very, very sad.

Later, the therapist discussed the patient's relationship with her boyfriend:

Therapist: Well, I'm not sure I understand completely; you've been going out with him for 15 years, and you act as if your realization that it is over is not significant.

Patient: I haven't been thinking about it. But I guess it is sad. I mean, my life is completely different now.

Therapist: In what way?

Patient: I'm not hanging around with any of the same people I usually do, but I'm still busy.

Therapist: It seems as if for some reason it's hard for you to admit the impact of this change.

Patient: [*Crying*] Yes, I guess it's much tougher than I thought. It's very sad, after all this time. Do you think these events were connected to my developing panic?

Therapist: Yes. Patients often experience losses preceding the onset of panic attacks. I feel that we need to understand more about the impact of these losses on you in order to help reduce your panic attacks.

Thus, early in treatment, the therapist made educational statements about panic disorder that were intended to reassure the patient about her symptoms and reduce her anxiety level. As in any psychodynamic treatment, however, the therapist's goals were to encourage the patient to explore the origins of her panic attacks on a psychological level.

Ms. G was using denial to defend against the emotional impact of recent losses in her life. The therapist demonstrated her denial with gentle confrontation, by questioning her about how she could be unaffected by the termination of a 15-year relationship. In this confrontation, the therapist invited Ms. G to become an observer of her own behavior, with the goal of increasing the patient's capacity for self-observation and her curiosity about herself. The meaning of the loss of her boyfriend and the memories of the deaths of her parents brought on by selling the house were overwhelming to Ms. G in a way that she had not clearly understood. Her panic attacks caused her to focus on her body and avoid the sadness and anger that she was experiencing with regard to these losses.

In Ms. G's case, therapy revealed evidence of ongoing characterological problems that made her vulnerable to the onset of panic. For example, the question of the factors that had led her to be involved in a problematic relationship for 15 years, and that had led to the realization at this point that it was not permanent, remained important foci for further exploration. The fact that Ms. G needed to deny her emotional states—causing her to have inadequate information about how she was reacting to stresses—also remained a chronic, characterological element in her predisposition to develop panic.

Ms. G's panic attacks resolved rapidly, and she became more curious about the origin of her current symptoms. Nevertheless, she terminated her treatment after 3 months of weekly psychotherapy in a panic-free state, although the therapist felt that, because of her long-standing style of managing her feelings, she could have benefited from a more extended period of psychotherapy.

Chapter 5

Psychodynamic Conflicts in Panic Disorder

By exploring the circumstances and feelings preceding panic onset, the therapist and the patient can develop a better understanding of the unconscious conflicts that are central in the genesis of the patient's panic disorder. Themes that emerge over time in therapy often involve conflicts about separation, anger, and sexuality. The therapist can help the patient elucidate how these conflicts lead to panic symptoms.

Separation and Independence

Clinical observations suggest that fantasies surrounding separation and independence are common areas of conflict for panic patients; several epidemiological studies provide indirect support for this finding. In the Yale Family Study, for example, Weissman et al. (1984) found that panic disorder in parents conferred more than a threefold risk of separation anxiety disorder in their children ages 6–17 years. Rosenbaum et al. (1988) found that 84.6% of the children of parents with panic disorder and agoraphobia demonstrated behavioral inhibition, a significantly greater frequency than a comparison group of children of persons with other psychiatric disorders. This risk may represent genetic or psychological vulnerability. In addition, retrospective studies of the childhood histories of adults and prospective studies of children at high risk for the development of anxiety disorders (where at least one parent has agoraphobia) suggest a relationship between separation anxiety disorder in childhood and subsequent agoraphobia in adulthood (Leonard and Rapoport 1989).

Patients commonly report that life events preceding the onset of panic disorder involve real or fantasized separation or loss from ambivalent objects. Panic thoughts typically involve fear of being alone and unable to care for oneself. Patients feel that they cannot survive alone; they often feel they need a phobic companion to protect against this and other dangers. This phenomenon is consistent with the well-known association between panic disorder and agoraphobia (American Psychiatric Association 1994; Freud 1895/1962, 1926/1950; Klein and Gorman 1987).

Psychodynamic psychotherapeutic treatment of panic disorder therefore must investigate the patient's intense fears of separation and the sense that he or she cannot function alone. These fears have their roots in childhood conflictual events and are connected to ongoing interpersonal difficulties. The early temperamental and emotional precursors—as described by Busch et al. (1991) and Shear et al. (1993)—set the stage for a separation-individuation process that is riddled with disappointments and conflicts, as well as future (later childhood and adult) difficulties with the modulation of anxiety and interpersonal intimacy.

These issues necessarily come to the fore in the patient's developing relationship with the therapist. Thus, many panic patients fear becoming "overly dependent" on their therapists, as they have with other important people in their lives. This outlook may manifest itself in the therapeutic situation in a variety of ways: patients frequently find the need to miss sessions or, at the other extreme, come too early and wait for hours before sessions. These fears may inhibit some patients' ability to become engaged in psychotherapy. Conversely, other patients may become quite dependent on the therapist; these patients may respond with mounting terror or intense sadness to changes in meeting times and therapist vacations. The therapeutic setting, by its nature, provides many natural inroads for the exploration and reemergence of this important set of conflicts.

Case Example

Ms. J, a 34-year-old woman, first developed panic disorder while driving herself from one city to another, en route to her 21st birthday party—which she had envisioned as her "final independence" from her mother. Before her first panic attack, she had been terrified and excited that this birthday meant that she had become an adult. During the initial panic attack, Ms. J had to pull off the road because she felt she was unable to continue driving. In her panic state, she telephoned her mother to come and pick her up; her mother refused, saying that Ms. J was able to drive herself and was just being silly.

For the next 8 years, Ms. J had multiple daily panic attacks; she was unable to go out alone, hold a job, or continue in school. In ironic contrast to her fantasy that her 21st birthday party symbolized her independence from her mother, this event ultimately marked the beginning of a total inability to function in the most basic ways without her mother.

Not surprisingly, when Ms. J entered psychotherapy years later, her conflicts about independence and intimacy immediately came to the fore. She frequently cancelled or forgot sessions. As in her relationship with her mother, Ms. J feared becoming dependent on the therapist; she worried that if she did, the therapist would not respond to her needs. One month after Ms. J began her treatment, the therapist addressed this issue.

Therapist: The last thing you want is for me to become important to you. I think you believe I'd never be there for you if that happened, and you'd be hurt.

Patient: You're right. Sometimes I feel it would kill me.

This interchange helped Ms. J understand her acting out and stimulated her to attend her sessions more regularly.

Anger

Clinical observations suggest that patients with panic disorder have intense difficulties tolerating and modulating their angry feelings and thoughts (Busch et al. 1991; Shear et al. 1993). Fear of angry feelings—along with conscious and unconscious vindictive fantasies that accompany these feelings—frequently triggers panic attacks. To facilitate exploration of angry constellations (and accompanying dangerous fantasies), the therapist must approach the patient in a nonjudgmental manner; the therapist must communicate to the patient that the dangers with which the patient is wrestling exist on a fantasy level. Some patients maintain that they are rarely, if ever, angry; these patients gradually become aware of their anger during the process of psychotherapy.

The family's management of anger may be informative. Familial difficulty with the management of rage or hostility may manifest itself in a variety of ways, including a history of family acrimony and violence. Furthermore, children may understand parental expression of anxiety as carrying the significance of an expression of rage. For example, parents often are consumed with fears about their children's well-being and safety at times when a child breaks a family rule (e.g., coming home late after curfew), which the child knows angers the parents. The patient may incorporate this unconscious childhood understanding of the often unstated significance of parental anxiety symptoms into fantasies about the meaning of the expression of his or her own rage and anxiety symptoms.

Conflicts relating to anger can impair the ability of panic patients to discuss their feelings and fantasies directly during treatment. Some patients who have observed uncontrollable anger in their parents have felt fear for their own safety. Understandably, these fears translate to the psychotherapeutic relationship, making the patient reluctant to express anger. The therapist must incorporate these historical factors into his or her understanding of the meaning of the patient's panic attacks, as well as the timing and structure of therapeutic interventions.

Panic patients commonly fantasize that rage or its expression will result in abandonment by the people on whom the patient most depends. Unconscious homicidal fantasies, conflicting with loving feelings, may be central in patients' difficulty with mastery of separation. These fears are not necessarily connected to actual experiences of childhood; they may represent compelling childhood fantasies.

Panic patients often exhibit inhibitions in discussing these topics in psychotherapy. Patients' fears of acknowledging angry feelings toward the therapist—who necessarily serves in the capacity of a model for important, conflicted relationships—may contribute to this reticence.

Case Example

Ms. K, a 35-year-old woman, presented for treatment of her second episode of panic disorder. A review of the history of her recurrent panic episodes indicated that conflicted—at times unconscious—rage at people she loved often preceded the onset of her symptoms.

Patient: In the fall, I felt like I had all the burdens to deal with for the family. My husband was particularly busy at that time, and he was never around to help me.

Therapist: How did you feel about that?

Patient: Overwhelmed at times. Particularly when he complained about something I did when he didn't even try to help me with the decision.

Therapist: Did that make you angry?

Patient: Yes, it did. And then, in addition to that, my mother was ill, and she and my brother expected me to take care of her. I don't see why I had to take care of her, particularly when my brother was closer to her. But I still felt I had to do it. I was infuriated about that as well.

Therapist: What happened then?

Patient: Well, I began to withdraw from them and felt increasingly alone and angry. I began to have anxious periods. When I was anxious, I didn't feel angry, just frightened. My son became an increasing burden. He clung to me instead of playing with other children. He kept waking me up at night, and I couldn't get a full night's rest.

Therapist: Were you angry at him as well?

Patient: Oh no. He's a child. He can't help it. But it did become frustrating.

Ms. K's first episode, which had occurred shortly after the birth of her son 4 years earlier, came at a time of similar stresses. Her husband, a prominent lawyer, was particularly busy with his work; she was struggling with the demands of her new baby; and her mother had been ill. Notably, although she denied being angry at her child, she regarded him as quite demanding; she said that his behavior was "frustrating." This pattern is typical of panic patients' struggle with angry feelings (see Chapter 6).

Consciously, Ms. K saw anger as a "waste": it accomplished nothing useful. This attitude was a rationalization to protect herself from the danger of her affects, as represented in violent fantasies. Ms. K feared that her anger was uncontrollable; she described a series of incidents in which she had either physically hurt people or feared that she would. For example, she had found herself brandishing a knife during a fight with her first husband. She said that her mother had reported "breaking her" of her anger in childhood, but she would not describe how this had been accomplished; she said she could not remember.

Ms. K described a pattern of "indignities" that triggered the rage that often preceded her panic episodes. Typically, these events entailed demands by others for Ms. K to take on unwanted chores or responsibilities—tasks that humiliated her. For example, she felt that her family unfairly demanded that she take care of her ill mother. Yet she felt guilty about being so angry, and she worried that her mother might die.

Exploration in psychotherapy revealed that these thoughts were related to "indignities" that Ms. K experienced at the hands of her mother early in life; her mother had become restrictive of her activities during her adolescence, after ignoring most of what she did as a child. When Ms. K became angry with her mother, her mother totally ignored her—leaving Ms. K feeling alone and abandoned.

During psychotherapy, Ms. K saw a connection between her anger and her panic attacks. She noticed that she began to have a limited-symptom panic attack after feeling increasingly angry with a colleague during an argument. An opportunity arose to explore these feelings in the transference; Ms. K felt angry that the therapist was not able to prevent her anxiety, which had increased to near-panic levels in the context of new stresses at home and work. The therapist told Ms. K that she was feeling abandoned by him and worried that he could not help her—just as she perceived her husband and others as uncaring and unable to help her. As Ms. K acknowledged her anger and reexperienced it in the therapeutic setting, her anxiety diminished, and she was able to be more assertive with her husband in seeking help in caring for their child.

Sexual Excitement

Although panic attacks often occur in the context of conflicted hostility, for some patients the attacks also take on a significance of their own—beyond the common, manifest panic thoughts of being ill and dying or becoming "crazy." In a number of our patients, the panic episodes themselves have a frightening and arousing inherent excitement, often closely tied to sadomasochistic sexual conflicts. These patients frequently present complaining about their panic attacks, yet they may be reluctant to be rid of them. Patients say that without the constant anxiety with which they have been living, life would seem "boring"; the attacks provide excitement and, for some, a distraction from more disturbing thoughts and fantasies.

Panic attacks, like any symptom, may take on various meanings in a patient's psychic economy. The patient cannot successfully relinquish these symptoms until he or she also grasps these secondary dynamic reinforcers of the symptoms and finds alternative methods to cope with these conflicts. If these dynamics are operative, patients in the therapeutic setting often unconsciously place themselves in "exciting" or arousing struggles with their therapists.

Case Example

Mr. L, a 19-year-old college student who had multiple daily panic episodes, kept himself close to a panic state at all times by drinking quarts of strong coffee. When the therapist explored this behavior, the patient reported that he "loved" the feeling of being so "wound up" that he was always close to a state of panic. "It's exciting," he said.

Mr. L became extremely anxious when he felt passive, "unmanly," or vulnerable. He had been sexually seduced by his mother in early childhood; his fear of passivity was closely connected to this history. Staying near an ultra-alert, panic state protected him from the disturbing, passive longings that his panic attacks themselves unconsciously represented.

Mr. L frequently initiated struggles with his therapist about who was in charge. Outwardly, Mr. L always wanted to be in control, even though he often begged "to be ordered" to do things, such as his homework. Initially, he had difficulty acknowledging this attitude; as often happens, however, the process that he experienced with others was easier for him to explore when it emerged in transference. An exchange in the second month of his treatment illustrates this dynamic.

Patient: Tell me what to talk about. I'm not going to talk about anything till you tell me what to say. I might talk about things that are unimportant, and waste my time here.

Therapist: It sounds like you want me to order you around so much that you won't even talk without my prior approval.

Patient: Well, I don't know what's important. You do. You just don't want to tell me.

Therapist: At the moment, what does seem clear is that you feel that I'm neglecting you, depriving you of my knowledge, and that you're angry at me. But it does seem that this whole process, of being in a struggle with me, happens over and over.

Patient: I know. [*Grins and giggles*]

Therapist: It seems like there's something a little fun about being in a fight with me.

Mr. L gradually realized that he found these struggles intensely exciting. He brought them about repeatedly, grinning and becoming physically jittery when they occurred. Exploring this patient's exciting need to try to provoke the therapist became important in Mr. L's efforts to relinquish his panic symptoms.

Case Example

Ms. M, a 27-year-old woman whose mother was a concentration camp survivor with an undiagnosed psychotic disorder, experienced panic attacks during fights with her boyfriend—whom she occasionally provoked into hitting her—as well as during sexual intercourse. As she became sexually excited, Ms. M had conscious fantasies of knocking her boyfriend unconscious with furniture. These thoughts routinely preceded her panic attacks.

During psychotherapy, Ms. M recognized that she experienced her boyfriend's sexual advances as physical attacks and that this feeling frightened but also aroused her; it kept her "on edge." Although Ms. M found her panic attacks frightening at times, they did not always bother her. When she presented for treatment, she did not think of the attacks as something she could—or even wanted to—change. "They're this crazy part of my life," she said. "They don't bother me."

Chapter 6

Defense Mechanisms in Panic Disorder

Patients' defense mechanisms are important in the treatment of panic disorder because of their role in anxiety management. Defense mechanisms are intrapsychic dynamisms that enable patients to avoid unconscious frightening affects and fantasies. In this chapter, we briefly review the most prominent defensive processes in panic patients, describe how these defenses may operate, and offer some guidance about how best to approach them in psychotherapy.

Panic patients may use any type of defense mechanism; clinical research and our own observations suggest, however, that these patients use certain defenses more frequently than others. Defense mechanisms commonly used by patients with panic disorder include reaction formation, undoing, and somatization (Andrews et al. 1989; Busch et al. 1995; Pollock and Andrews 1989). In addition, we have found that patients frequently use the defense of externalization, similar to the way they focus on their bodies (somatization).

Reaction Formation

Reaction formation is a defense mechanism in which an affect is disguised as its opposite. For example, rage may appear as an excessive amount of caring or concern, or a romantic attachment may manifest as "hating" or criticism. Panic patients frequently exhibit reaction formation as an unconscious mechanism; it solidifies the tie to a significant other at a time when the patient experiences that tie as being threatened by anger.

When a panic patient incongruously raises how positively or negatively he or she feels about someone, the therapist should evaluate whether reaction formation is present: the patient may be unconsciously masking the opposite set of feelings. Therapy can fruitfully address these feelings. The following case example demonstrates how psychotherapy can successfully monitor reaction formation to help patients gain further control over their lives.

Case Example

Mr. N was a 26-year-old man who presented with a 9-year history of panic disorder; during the periods of his most extreme symptomatology, Mr. N had seven to eight panic attacks per day. The attacks were intense experiences for him because he had the sensation that he was suffocating. Although Mr. N's panic attacks were brief, between attacks he remained quite anxious, without autonomic symptoms, and he had an almost constant sense of foreboding that "something really scary" might happen. This "scary thing" remained undefined, although it seemed to be connected vaguely with the possibility that Mr. N might hurt someone else.

Mr. N had grown up on a large farm in a western state. At age 17 years—after the sudden death of his best male friend caused by a cerebral aneurysm—Mr. N had joined the Air Force. He had served in the military for 4 years and was involved in active combat overseas, although he did not fire a weapon during his combat experiences. While Mr. N was in the Air Force, he began to self-medicate for his extreme anxiety—first with heavy alcohol use and later with marijuana and benzodiazepines, which he obtained illegally.

By the time Mr. N presented for treatment, he was physically dependent on high doses of alprazolam and was using marijuana daily, although he had stopped consuming alcohol. Despite this regimen, he continued to have a constant sense of foreboding, and he experienced several panic attacks per week. Mr. N was consciously frightened of his anger. When he presented, he told his therapist, "My terror of getting angry makes no rational sense because I've never hurt anyone. I don't even think I've been in a fight since high school."

At the time of presentation, Mr. N was breaking off a 2-year relationship with his fiancee. He initially described his reasons for doing so as, "We're just wrong for each other. I love her as a person, but I'm just not attracted to her anymore." Over the first several weeks of psychotherapy, however, Mr. N gradually revealed that he was locked in a raging, high-stakes battle with his fiancee, her friends, and her family. Although he could describe the events clearly, he seemed to be unaware that a battle was taking place at all. He was extremely reluctant to acknowledge any angry feelings toward his girlfriend, although he had ample objective reasons to be enraged.

Mr. N reluctantly told his therapist that his girlfriend had stolen several thousand dollars from him—money he had been painstakingly saving from a variety of different jobs to put himself through his senior year of college. Interestingly, Mr. N believed that feeling any anger about this turn of events might be "unfair and chauvinist"; his response at the time he had discovered the theft had been, "Oh, well, she really needed the money, and she's much younger (4 years) than I am. I can't reasonably hold her responsible. She's not a mature person."

At a time when Mr. N should have been reevaluating how much he could trust his girlfriend, he found himself unaccountably compelled to give her more money for other things that she needed. In addition, for the first time in their stormy relationship, he allowed his girlfriend to hit him.

In therapy, Mr. N gradually explored this reaction formation and the unconscious rage at his girlfriend that it symbolized. He also uncovered violent fantasies about mutilating his girlfriend in retaliation—fantasies he was trying to ignore (and which made him describe himself as "chauvinist"). This process was central in enabling Mr. N finally to disengage himself from what had been a masochistic relationship, 4 months after starting therapy. This exploration also helped him to stop smoking marijuana and to gain more control over his anxiety symptoms.

Undoing

Undoing serves a similar purpose to reaction formation: to reassure the patient (and the individual on whom he or she feels dependent) that any negative affect that becomes conscious or is expressed has been retracted and disavowed. The use of undoing presents an opportunity for therapists to point out to patients how negative affects often must be disavowed immediately. This awareness can help patients acknowledge the intensity of their discomfort with the feelings they are tentatively expressing.

Case Example

Ms. K (see Chapter 5) frequently used the defense mechanism of undoing.

Patient: I got to where I really hated my husband—and believe me, I really love him.

Therapist: I notice that whenever you describe your anger at your husband, you then say how much you love him. It's as if you are reassuring yourself.

Patient: Yes, you've mentioned that pattern before, and now I'm beginning to see what you mean. I guess I'm less comfortable with my anger at him than I thought I was.

The therapist had pointed out on several previous occasions Ms. K's tendency to make a comment that served to undo her anger. Over time, she became aware that this was her pattern and that it was an important clue to her degree of ambivalence. This realization allowed Ms. K to examine her experience of anger at the point at which she felt the urge to undo it. She learned that she became anxious and guilty after expressing anger, fearing that others would see her as a "bad girl" and reject her; that fear then caused her to become inhibited, submissive, and frustrated that she had not expressed herself in the way she wanted. Ms. K's increasing knowledge about her feelings and behavior helped her to feel safer experiencing and expressing her angry feelings.

Somatization and Externalization

Because panic patients tend to somatize rather than acknowledge inner feeling states, they often have extreme difficulty with the process of looking inward. This problem may be an inherent aspect of patients' defensive styles—the same defensive styles that give rise to panic attacks. By focusing on bodily concerns (somatization) and the problems of others (externalization), panic patients attempt to avoid addressing emotional states and conflicts. The therapist must address these defenses when they arise in psychotherapy.

Examples of somatization appear throughout this book. For example, Ms. C (see Chapter 4) focused on actual experiences of suffocation; she scratched her skin to avoid direct feelings of suffocation and rage that she experienced with her mother. Ms. G (see Chapter 4) experienced shortness of breath, rather than thinking of the painful memories of her mother's demise. Although these patients initially did not see the connection between their feelings and their symptoms, they began to understand those connections during the initial weeks of therapy.

In cases of externalization, panic patients commonly begin their treatment by focusing entirely on the problems of others. Initially, the therapist may choose to let the patient continue to discuss other people, looking for patterns in the way the patient views others. The therapist can then encourage the patient to look at his or her own role in relationships with other people. If the patient persists in focusing on other people's problems and anxieties, the therapist can point out that the patient seems to feel more comfortable focusing on others and invite the patient to explore this pattern. The therapist can then make a connection between the patient's own anxiety and that of the patient's friends; alternatively, the therapist may point out that talking about other people's anxieties makes the patient feel less anxious, and therefore stronger, in psychotherapy—where he or she presumably is frightened. The clinical data and the intensity of the patient's need to deny the severity of symptoms should determine which technique the therapist chooses.

Case Example

O, a 13-year-old girl with panic disorder and an elevator phobia, begged her mother to enroll her in psychotherapy for her symptoms. Although O's problems were long-standing, she was beginning to feel that being so frightened so frequently was becoming more difficult. Nonetheless, after describing her symptoms in detail in the first session of her psychotherapy, O seemed to be unwilling to return to the topic of her phobia or her panic attacks. Instead, she spent her sessions discussing her friends' problems in detail. In particular, she focused on the anxiety symptoms of H, a close female friend. O described her friend's fears as "stupid" but occasionally added that she too knew what it was like to be irrational. The following exchange occurred during the second month of twice weekly psychotherapy.

Therapist: I wonder if you've noticed that you often tell me about H's problems.

Patient: Yeah, I guess I do. But she seems like such an idiot, worrying about these stupid things.

Therapist: I'm beginning to think that maybe you feel like there's something "stupid" or shameful about the problems you're having. Maybe you've been telling me about H's problems because they remind you of some of the difficulties that brought you to see me.

Patient: I dunno. Maybe.

Because of the urgency that panic patients experience during panic episodes themselves, many of these patients need to prove to themselves and everyone else—including their therapists—that they are indeed strong and capable. Discussing others often is a relief. As we noted in Chapter 4, many panic patients view their anxiety symptoms as deeply humiliating.

Offering too many interpretations about others reinforces externalization, thereby aggravating the difficulty with inward exploration. The therapist may encourage the patient to refer to a "part" of himself or herself feeling hurt or angry, as Anna Freud pointed out (J. Sandler et al. 1980). This useful technique helps to emphasize the idea that intrapsychic conflicts are responsible for the production of symptoms. Another maneuver would involve a statement about the conflictual nature of wishes: "You are afraid of your wish to injure or sexually use or hit or murder; therefore, you need to talk about others struggling with these feelings."

Chapter 7

Transference, Working Through, and Termination

Working With Transference

In the course of psychotherapy, the panic patient's conflicts in relationships become focused on the person of the therapist, allowing for more direct exploration. In this context, unconscious fantasies that underlie panic attacks emerge. Transference is a powerful tool that allows the patient to reexperience affective states and fantasized relationships within the confines of the therapeutic dyad and explore conflicts within the safe framework of psychotherapy.

Careful focus on transference is a central therapeutic element in the practice of psychodynamic psychotherapy, and proper work in this arena can help in reducing the patient's vulnerability to the recurrence of panic episodes. The occurrence of pre-panic states, limited-symptom attacks, or full-blown panic attacks in the psychotherapeutic setting may help the therapist identify highly specific triggers of panic that otherwise are inaccessible to the patient.

Transference provides a powerful view of the patient's unconscious fantasy life. The therapist therefore must carefully avoid unnecessarily influencing the nature of transference with issues the therapist brings into the treatment setting; furthermore, the therapist must remain as professional and nonjudgmental as possible. Even if a patient's fears and phobic concerns sound extremely unrealistic, the therapist should treat them as real concerns; the fantasies that underlie these fears are based on some core historical reality that must be explored and understood, not merely dismissed.

Many extremely anxious patients attempt to engage their therapists actively in the decision-making difficulties with which they struggle, thereby relieving themselves of the anxiety that accompanies decision making. Therapists must avoid the pitfall of giving advice, however. The goal of psychotherapy is to help patients make their own decisions and to understand why decisions are so anxiety-provoking—not to take over the executive functions of running the patients' lives for them.

Patients have real reactions to therapists as real people. Even "real" reactions, however, are influenced by underlying unconscious fantasies, which the patient must understand. The therapist should stay alert to the patient's feelings and fantasies about the treatment and the therapist, as they arise.

The nature of the patient's comfort in describing his or her reactions to the treatment situation and to the therapist determines how rapidly and directly the therapist can address transference. Skirting the topic for too long or missing a patient's cues may reinforce the patient's fears that negative feelings about the therapist are intolerable for the therapist—just as the patient often perceives his or her parents' reactions to these feelings. Therefore, the therapist should make transference analogies whenever possible.

However, a panic patient may perceive early, aggressive focus by the therapist on transference as an attack or intrusion; the patient may meet transference with denial and anger if the therapist pursues it too vigorously. If a patient becomes angry or anxious when the therapist touches on the patient's feelings about the therapist, the therapist should point out this phenomenon to the patient before making further transference observations. This process often leads to valuable insights about the patient's resistance to examining transference. It also will reflect the patient's problems with other significant relationships in his or her life.

Some panic patients manage intense feelings about the therapist by never mentioning them or by not permitting themselves to experience such feelings at all—similar to the way they manage other intense feelings. This type of emotional backdrop can foster somatization as a way to avoid psychic distress. These patients may experience intense transference; if the therapist allows the patient to avoid exploring these issues throughout the course of the treatment, this intense transference can interfere with the reduction of panic vulnerability.

Even if the therapist can easily observe displacement from transference in the patient's description of another relationship, the therapist may pursue interpretations by focusing on the extra-therapeutic relationship until the patient can more readily discuss his or her feelings about the therapist. Another approach in this type of situation focuses on the patient's reticence: the therapist may observe to the patient that "One thing we know is that you don't wish to admit to any feelings about me at all."

Case Example

Ms. P, a 24-year-old woman with panic disorder, frequently came to therapy sessions feeling upset and hurt by one of a group of girlfriends whom she wanted to impress. Ms. P cited many instances in these relationships in which she felt she had been slighted; in her fantasy, these slights often were purposeful.

In psychotherapy, Ms. P frequently appeared to feel slighted by her therapist as well. Issues regarding the timing of sessions, or the fact that her therapist once had been 5 minutes late for a meeting, reinforced this fantasy. Ms. P did not openly express her feelings of hurt, however. Instead, she made inadvertent comments to the therapist about the physician's "busyness" and how she thought she was in the way. On several occasions when the therapist directly pointed out Ms. P's asides, Ms. P denied feeling hurt by the therapist; each time, however, she seemed quite irritated that the therapist had mentioned the subject. The following exchange occurred at the end of the ninth month of psychotherapy.

Patient: This really has nothing to do with you; it's just me, the way I talk.

Therapist: You seem set against our even thinking about why you've been telling me that you feel like your problems are in my way.

Patient: Well, it's just my stuff. It's irrational, I guess. Anyway, it's embarrassing.

Therapist: How come?

Patient: [*Crying*] I just feel so beholden to you and kind of dependent on you. I told myself that I'd never let myself get like that. How could I mean anything to you in the way our relationship means so much to me? Sometimes I feel that I just live from session to session, but at the end of our 50 minutes, you just leave and go live your life, and I'm left hanging on.

Therapist: Why do you think it's been so hard to talk about this? I know that you think it's important.

Patient: I just feel I'll lose you altogether if I don't keep some of this to myself.

We review this case in greater depth at the end of this volume (see Chapter 11). This case highlights how a therapist can use a patient's transference to help him or her to alter habitual views and actions with others in psychotherapy.

Working Through

Working through is a gradual process in which patients steadily apply their acquired knowledge of their conflicts and psychic functioning to increase their understanding of the ways these conflicts affect other areas of their lives. This phase is helpful in reducing the patient's vulnerability to panic recurrence; in the process of working through, the patient explores contributing factors to this vulnerability.

In the psychotherapeutic situation, the process is marked by the need for a specific interpretation to be repeated in different contexts as it applies to different manifestations of the same intrapsychic phenomenon. In this way, patients begin to appreciate how this particular set of dynamics has affected them. Patients typically demonstrate improved functioning in work and relationships as they become more conscious of how their conflicts affect various areas of their lives.

The therapist must be aware that panic patients rarely change significantly in response to a single interpretation—no matter how central—and that the success or failure of a line of interpretive work depends on how the therapist prepares the patient for the interpretation, as well as how the therapist handles the working through phase. In addition, an interpretation may be rephrased and modified by the patient, who brings it into closer approximation with his or her experience. However, a negative response to an interpretation may not signify that it is incorrect; the patient simply may not be ready to hear the new formulation. Nonetheless, the therapist should note the patient's response and reconsider the interpretation or formulation, if necessary.

Patients with panic disorder—by the nature of their symptomatic profile—have inherent difficulty connecting their often overwhelming feelings with intellectually understandable ideas. As a consequence, the working through process may be prolonged and marked by difficulties making connections among different aspects of life. Furthermore, the therapist must determine what constitutes sufficient working through of a particular phenomenon. The therapist should base this determination on whether the working through process has sufficiently reinforced the change created by the interpretation and whether that change will break down under predictable stress. The therapist should assess the patient's awareness of the nature of panic triggers and the patient's ability to manage effectively the challenges brought up in these situations.

Working through occurs outside the therapeutic setting as well as in therapy sessions, as patients ponder what has transpired in treatment and recognize how it applies to their lives. For patients with panic disorder—who frequently perceive themselves as disempowered, passive, or helpless during their panic episodes—the working through process often involves a recognition of their passivity and dependence on others; these patients can gradually master their panic by learning to take more active care of themselves. In addition, panic patients often become increasingly aware of displaced or disavowed angry feelings during the course of psychotherapy. Increasing awareness and comfort with these feelings can lead to more direct and effective interactions with other people.

Case Example

At the end of the vignette in Chapter 5, Ms. K recognized a connection between her anger and her panic attacks after becoming angry with her therapist. This realization enabled her to be more direct and assertive with her husband.

Despite this early foray into assertiveness, however, Ms. K continued to be uncomfortable with anger in many situations. Most prominently, she felt conflicted about acknowledging and managing her anger at her mother. She noticed that she began to panic when she visited with her mother, so she avoided her mother entirely and did not speak to her for several weeks. Although Ms. K did not experience anxiety during the time she avoided her mother, she did feel guilty and concerned about her mother's medical condition.

When she visited her mother again, Ms. K was intensely uncomfortable; she recognized her feelings as those that routinely preceded her panic episodes. Ms. K's mother complained about Ms. K's recent absence and appeared ill. Ms. K had recognized in the past that her mother purposefully avoided taking proper care of herself when she felt mistreated, which led to recurrent bouts of her medical illness; Ms. K's guilt led her to take care of her mother even more at these times, which further intensified her unconscious anger and anxiety because she resented her mother's dependence on her. Nonetheless, in this instance Ms. K was not aware of feeling angry at her mother, and she did not confront her mother about not taking care of herself.

The therapist interpreted Ms. K's unacknowledged anger on several occasions, comparing it with anger she had experienced in other situations and now was able to recognize. Ms. K responded that she knew she must be angry at her mother because at other times her mother's behavior infuriated her. In this episode, however, Ms. K did not experience any anger, and she felt frustrated.

Ms. K then recalled an incident in which her mother had called the wife of Ms. K's married lover to inform the woman about Ms. K's affair with her husband. Ms. K told her therapist she had felt "stunned" rather than angry when she found out about her mother's actions; she had never been able to discuss the episode with her mother. Revisiting this incident in therapy, Ms. K recognized the audacity of her mother's intrusiveness—which she believed was common for her mother—and slowly acknowledged the murderous rage she had felt in response to similar intrusions at other times.

Ms. K recognized that her sense of being "stunned" made her feel confused and also served as a protective device so that she would be unable to acknowledge her anger or hurt her mother. The process of working through allowed Ms. K to recognize that she was angry at her mother in the current situation as well and enabled her to confront her mother about her manipulative behavior.

Termination

Panic patients frequently have significant conflicts concerning issues of loss, separation, and independence. These highly charged subjects frequently are a focus of exploration in psychodynamic psychotherapy with panic patients; separations from significant others arise repeatedly as precipitants of panic attacks. In the transference, panic patients may perceive empathic failures by the therapist as abandonments; these feelings bring this set of conflicts to the fore. Therapist vacations, as well as the time between sessions, provide opportunities to explore patients' reactions to separations.

An important aspect of working through feelings concerning separation focuses on the patient's ability to experience rage at the object involved—without becoming so threatened that separation becomes impossible. This issue is particularly difficult for panic patients; it requires working through repeated experiences of separation. Despite an unavoidable focus on these issues throughout the course of therapy, the termination phase of treatment with panic patients often involves an intensification of feelings of hurt and abandonment, as well as anger at the therapist. Thus, termination provides a crucial opportunity to solidify gains in the development of the patient's sense of maturity, independence, and competence.

Some patients may wish to terminate treatment after the resolution of a panic episode. Although such separation may be appropriate in certain cases, panic patients commonly require further work to prevent the recurrence of symptoms. Patients may be afraid to address underlying affects and conflicts that remain unconscious during panic episodes. For panic patients in particular—with their conflicts over intimacy, independence, and separation—the recommendation to establish a long-term, psychotherapeutic relationship can be particularly frightening. Panic patients often terminate treatment precipitously, only to return after a recurrence of panic symptoms.

Case Example

Mr. Q experienced a resolution of panic symptoms after three sessions of psychodynamic psychotherapy. In subsequent sessions, he began to explore conflicts with his intrusive mother and his difficulties with angry feelings that were central to the onset of his panic attacks. Mr. Q continued to have significant difficulties in his relationships, particularly with women, and tended to isolate himself rather than become closer to other people and risk potential rejection.

After 12 additional sessions, Mr. Q expressed a desire to discontinue therapy. The therapist stated that although Mr. Q's panic symptoms had resolved, his tendency to isolate himself led to feelings of loneliness that in turn made him particularly vulnerable to panic recurrence.

Indeed, when Mr. Q attempted to become involved in a more intimate relationship, he became frightened. He did not know why this happened.

The therapist suggested that Mr. Q needed to explore further what prevented him from becoming more intimately involved with others. The therapist believed that these fears were precisely what made continued treatment seem unpleasant. After some thought, Mr. Q agreed to continue treatment.

Mr. Q's therapy continued for another 8 months; during that time, he had no recurrence of panic attacks or episodes of intense anxiety, and he gradually was able to permit himself to become more involved with others. Despite this progress, however, Mr. Q still shied away from intense intimacy.

Case Example

Ms. P (see earlier and Chapter 11) had been in psychotherapy three times each week for 3 years when she began to think about ending her treatment. The panic attacks she had presented with had resolved entirely within 2 months of the beginning of her treatment. Ms. P had spent the remainder of her time in psychotherapy exploring several thorny issues: a desperate yet ambivalent desire to become involved in a relationship with a man; conflicts about becoming more independent from her family; rage at her rigid, somewhat perverse, and unpredictable father; and mixed feelings about taking on a more self-sufficient role. The latter conflict often interfered with her professional functioning in graduate school. All of these issues had contributed, to a certain extent, to Ms. P's anxiety symptoms.

In the transference, Ms. P's relationship with her therapist had dramatically altered over the course of the psychotherapy. Ms. P initially had taken a childlike, dependent attitude toward the therapist—treating the therapist as though she were perfect and actively complaining that the therapist should provide more structure and care for Ms. P's life. This relationship strongly resembled the patient's description of her relationship to her mother (when her mother was alive); Ms. P continued to have a similarly structured relationship with her sister (who often took a mothering role with Ms. P).

As Ms. P's autonomous functioning improved during psychotherapy, her transference evolved, and she began to perceive the therapist as more critical. Ms. P had the fantasy—which she recognized as unrealistic—that the therapist did not want her to move away emotionally by establishing a romantic relationship with a man. Ms. P found herself enraged at the therapist over these issues; although she was able to explore the connection between these fantasies and fantasies she must have had about her mother when she was alive, Ms. P's anger at her therapist often felt quite compelling.

In anticipation of her graduation from graduate school, Ms. P began seriously to consider leaving the city. She offered many reasons, but the most intense and conflicted justification involved the fantasy that if she were to leave her treatment and "escape" her therapist, she would establish a relationship with a man. Although Ms. P recognized the unrealistic nature of this fantasy, she aggressively pursued a job opportunity in a distant city; during the therapist's 1-week vacation, Ms. P agreed to take the job on an emergency basis. As she told her therapist about her decision after the vacation, Ms. P became extremely anxious and tearful and felt trapped into going to her new job.

Although the contract Ms. P had signed for the new job did not permit her to alter her decision, she almost immediately desperately wanted to do so. The therapist pointed out that she must have arranged this situation to "make" herself go, given how conflicted and frightened she felt about leaving the therapist.

Nevertheless, Ms. P arranged to delay beginning her new job by 1 year; she spent the time in therapy discussing her long-standing fears of independence and contrasting those fears with her growing awareness of her own competence and talents. "It's like I've spent my whole life avoiding these things about myself so I wouldn't ever have to sever any attachments," she commented, adding, "But I know I don't need to be in babyish relationships like that anymore."

In her last few months in the city, Ms. P began a sexual relationship with a man—something she had not permitted herself to do before. She acknowledged that this new relationship helped to diffuse the intensity of her preoccupation with leaving her therapist. Nonetheless, the relationship itself represented a real and important achievement in the life of this restricted young woman.

As the termination of therapy approached, Ms. P became more nostalgic about her treatment. She arranged to go to the new city to set up her apartment, but she saw her therapist several times on a return trip. "I feel like I'm taking a little bit of you with me," Ms. P remarked, "by coming back and telling you about my new life without you."

Despite fears that she would be miserable and lonely (and miss her therapist), Ms. P negotiated a successful move. During the following year, she wrote the therapist several long letters about her new life. Ms. P has not had a recurrence of her panic attacks in the 8 years since the termination of her treatment and she has been able to negotiate her professional and romantic life in a much more mature and successful way.

Chapter 8

Techniques of Psychodynamic Psychotherapy as They Apply to Panic Disorder

Working With Dreams and Other Fantasy Material

In his early work, Freud referred to dreams as the "royal road to the unconscious" (Freud 1900/1953, vol. 5, p. 608). Although psychiatrists currently debate the centrality of the use of dreams in psychoanalytic treatment as the most unalloyed expression of patients' central unconscious fantasies, dreams continue to be a valuable source of information about patients' unconscious fantasy lives.

Patients with panic disorder often have a propensity to somatize and disavow their emotional states and impulses. For these patients, dreams can take on a central significance in the therapeutic unraveling of the meaning of symptoms. Although a complete description of the technique of dream analysis is beyond the scope of this book, the following case example illustrates how a dream may be instrumental in revealing important fantasies about a patient's intrapsychic life.

Case Example

R, a 14-year-old eighth grader, presented with acute onset of severe panic disorder with agoraphobia; her symptoms prevented her from being alone even for a few minutes. R had been troubled by a recurrent dream, which she brought to the attention of the therapist during the second week of her twice weekly psychodynamic treatment. In the dream, R saw herself climbing up an endless ladder that seemed to be precariously placed over a cliff or abyss. Her mother was above her on the ladder, and R was aware of her mother's skirt brushing her face in an irritating way. R could not see much because of the skirt, and she was terrified.

R associated to the dream over several sessions, at a time when she again had the dream. R said that before the onset of her panic symptoms, her mother had frequently made her feel confined or stifled because of unreasonable anxieties about the dangers of the city. In particular, her mother would cite what R felt were simply excuses about transportation to object to R's attendance at coed parties.

Therapist: Why do you think they're just excuses?

Patient: Because she never does that when I have to travel around the city with my girlfriends. It's ridiculous. She's constantly lecturing me that I'm going to get pregnant! I don't even have a boyfriend, but she's been saying this to me since I was 12.

Therapist: How come?

Patient: I dunno. I guess since I got my period. It's totally retarded; she treats me like I'm from her stupid culture where girls get pregnant when they're my age. [*R's mother was an Hispanic immigrant.*] But I'm not from her culture; I'm from here! She just doesn't get it.

Therapist: You talk as though there's something about her culture that you object to.

Patient: I dunno, it's OK; just there are some stupid things about it, like this thing with women. They lose their brains around men. It's disgusting! I'm American. I could never be like that.

Therapist: In the dream, you're stuck on this scary ladder, following your mother. Have you ever had the thought that there's something about your mother's behavior with men that upsets you?

Patient: No, I don't think so. [*At this point, R became thoughtful and preoccupied throughout the rest of the session.*]

In the next session, R again seemed preoccupied and talked about being angry with her mother. Toward the end of the session, R made a slip about her half-sister's age, which embarrassed her. On exploration, R revealed that the embarrassing thing about the slip was that it betrayed her knowledge that her parents had been having an affair while her father had been married to his first wife—and that R owed her own existence to her mother's failure to use adequate contraception during this relationship.

This case example highlights how a central unconscious fantasy (here, the patient's unconscious, conflictual identification with her mother's sexual mores as she enacted them in the events leading to the patient's conception) can be contained in a dream. Careful exploration of the dream can provide the patient with an opportunity to learn more about the patient's unconscious conflicts and fantasies.

Clarification and Confrontation

Clarification and confrontation represent techniques in which the therapist brings feelings, thoughts, and behaviors to the attention of the patient. According to Greenson (1967), confrontation involves making psychic phenomena evident to the patient's conscious ego, and clarification aims at placing psychic phenomena in sharp focus. However, confrontations and clarifications cannot always be sharply differentiated.

Clarification enlists the observing ego of the patient to gain distance and a degree of objectivity toward the experiencing ego. Clarification also lays the groundwork for interpretation. For example, a therapist may point out that the patient always talks about terminating the treatment before the therapist's vacations. In another situation, a therapist might remark that the patient is no longer a helpless child—and that the patient's helpless, powerless image of himself or herself therefore is a distortion of reality, in accordance with long-lasting childhood feelings and fantasies.

According to Bibring (1954),

> Clarification . . . does . . . not refer to unconscious (repressed or otherwise warded off) material but to conscious and/or preconscious processes, of which the patient is not sufficiently aware, which escape his attention but which he recognizes more or less readily when they are clearly presented to him. . . . Clarification in therapy aims at those vague and obscure factors (frequently below the level of verbalization) which are relevant from the viewpoint of treatment; it refers to those techniques and

> therapeutic processes which assist the patient to reach a higher degree of self-awareness, clarity and differentiation of self-observation which makes adequate verbalization possible. (p. 755)

Thus, clarification is a necessary tool in the psychotherapeutic approach by which the patient gains an objective view of himself or herself; it also can be essential in understanding the patient's childhood history.

For patients with panic disorder, these techniques often are extremely useful in psychotherapeutic work to focus on the panic symptoms themselves. Panic patients frequently perceive normal physical variations (i.e., feeling hot, cold, or hungry) as signs of underlying illness or disease. They easily confuse their fantasies that they are sick and desperately in need of help with reality. Clarifications about emotional states as the source of physical sensations are almost universally essential in the treatment of panic patients.

Case Example

Mr. L (see Chapter 5) frequently told his therapist that he believed he was ill because of myriad tiny physical sensations. His complaints often related to how hot, cold, or hungry he was or how well he remembered barely studied course material. Mr. L often became frightened about intermittent abdominal pain, which seemed to be associated with irregular bowel habits. He construed ghastly implications from minimal alterations in his body; he believed that he had lead poisoning, Lyme disease, and AIDS all at the same time. Internists had assured him, however, that he was in robust physical health. The following exchange occurred during the fourth month of treatment.

Patient: I know you probably think I'm crazy, but last night I was thinking that I'm sure that there's lead in the water in my apartment. It's possible, you know. All the problems in my life could be due to lead poisoning.

Therapist: Of course, it's possible that there's lead in the water, but the fact is that you seem to prefer to assign frightening interpretations to your physical sensations rather than to think about how anxious you've been since exams began.

Patient: I know I do that. But the point is, I could be sick too. I could be in treatment for years for my emotions when really it's lead poisoning. I know my doctor said I'm fine, but it's hard to believe.

Therapist: Reality doesn't carry as much weight for you as your scary fantasies do. Also, you know that you always feel frightened about trusting people. You feel that about your internist and also about me, here. But the truth is that when you get particularly anxious, your assumption is that the feelings you're having are physical.

Patient: Yeah. I wonder why I do that. Actually, if I spent any time thinking about how much work I have left to do in the next three days, I'd completely lose it. I'm really in danger of getting F's this time.

Successful clarifications and confrontations do not preclude additional analysis of the patient's fantasies. They help the patient feel less threatened by terrifying misperceptions, thereby facilitating more detailed exploration. In Mr. L's case, the patient began to explore his sense of physical vulnerability (which had arisen following a childhood sexual seduction) only after the therapist pointed out his fear of trusting people in positions of authority and his need to see his problems as being "physical."

Significant Interpretations

Interpretations appear to be *significant* when changes in symptoms, behavior, or therapeutic process emerge subsequently. For patients with panic disorder, the number and severity of panic attacks often fluctuate with events in the course of treatment; therapists therefore must monitor symptoms closely during the course of psychotherapy.

However, the therapist may not always discern which portion of the interpretation the patient is responding to—or even what, precisely, the patient has heard the therapist say. Patients' paraphrased repetitions of what they believe the therapist has said often differ in many ways from what the therapist believes he or she has said. These differences often relate to the intense transferential and countertransferential overlay that develops between therapist and patient in the psychotherapeutic setting (see Jacobs 1986).

Changes occurring as a result of significant interpretations do not necessarily arise immediately subsequent to the interpretation. This delay makes assessing the efficacy of any given interpretation complex. A period in which the therapist restates the interpretation in different contexts and ways often is essential. Moreover, much important interpretive work precedes significant interpretations; this work makes such interpretations possible.

When a significant interpretation is successful, it facilitates a process whereby the patient recaptures early memories, affects, or fantasies relevant to the childhood experiences that are operative in the patient's current situation and connects the transference with genetic conflicts. Following an interpretation, the therapist may observe changes in the elaborated material that the patient brings to treatment, the flow of associations that the patient reports, or the patient's expression of symptoms. For panic patients, significant interpretations often affect the frequency or number of symptoms during panic attacks.

Case Example

A young woman, Ms. S, experienced panic attacks when she was enraged with her boyfriend; her symptoms were associated with thoughts that she needed his help and that he was not helping her because he was mean and did not care. The therapist had explored this interplay over a series of sessions. The patient's panic attacks had grown more frequent and disturbing in the month since she had entered treatment. (Exacerbation of symptoms in the early course of therapy does not necessarily mean that the treatment is failing; it may simply indicate that the therapeutic relationship is intensifying and that the patient's conflicts, which give rise to panic, are emerging in therapy.)

Therapist: So, what occurs to you about how much worse your panic attacks have become since you started coming to see me last month?

Patient: I don't know. This is the worst I've ever been in my life. Doesn't say too much about the treatment, huh? [*Laughing*]

Therapist: You know, I think that's a very important point. I think you feel I don't care about you and I don't want to, or can't, help you—just like you've been telling me you feel about your fiance. I think you've been feeling as furious at me as you have at him. It's very uncomfortable for you, having such mixed feelings about me. That's why your panic attacks are so bad now.

Patient: [*Laughing*] It's you! You're my problem! I guess this is really interesting. I don't know what to think about this.

Ms. S seemed to gain insight into an important dynamic mechanism involved in her panic attacks only when the therapist offered the interpretation that her panic attacks were worse since she entered treatment because she was enraged at the therapist and felt that the therapist "didn't care and was not helping." Ms. S's panic attacks disappeared subsequent to this session; over the next several sessions, she began to produce a flood of childhood memories of panic attacks in which she had felt alone and terrified—in particular when she was with her older sister, who physically abused Ms. S when their parents were out.

Many patients find one interpretation to be particularly important. They may return to it repeatedly in different settings, as Ms. S did with the therapist's interpretation about getting worse in treatment because she felt neglected by the therapist.

Chapter 9

Approaches to Common Problems in the Treatment of Panic Patients

Phobic Companions

A patient with a phobic companion may perceive the therapist as an intruder into the patient's intense, conflicted relationship with the phobic companion. For these patients, the therapist and the treatment itself represent a real threat to the exclusiveness and closeness of this important, albeit ambivalent, relationship (Deutsch 1929). When this problem is particularly severe, therapeutic work may be impossible until the patient can achieve some separation from the phobic companion. Often, the phobic companion must be included in initial sessions; this early phase of treatment involves working toward gradual separation.

Case Example

Mr. T, an 18-year-old high school graduate, presented for treatment after 1½ years of progressive physical weakness and social isolation, as well as consuming anxiety that he was going to die of a physical disease (although extensive and ongoing medical workups had produced negative results); in comparison, his frequent panic attacks and severe anticipatory anxiety were minor. An honor roll student from an extremely competitive high school, Mr. T was preparing to enter a prestigious university far from home when his weakness became so severe that he was confined to bed, unable even to feed himself or use the bathroom. Furthermore, Mr. T was unable to function without one of his parents, even for brief periods, without becoming acutely anxious. Consequently, Mr. T's father felt compelled to leave his job to care for his son.

When Mr. T began his twice weekly treatment, he presented in a wheelchair, propelled by his father. He and his parents were terrified and skeptical about the idea of psychotherapy. Moreover, they would not allow Mr. T to meet with the therapist alone: Both parents attended all sessions, and neither Mr. T nor his parents would accept the therapist's suggestion that the parents wait outside the office.

Initially, the entire family seemed to defend the status quo, however difficult it appeared to be. During therapy sessions, for example, Mr. T's mother repeatedly interrupted the conversation to ask whether he was too warm and needed her to take off his jacket for him. Moreover, Mr. T seemed to be quite reluctant to talk about his feelings; when the conversation began to focus on feelings, he frequently changed the subject to the more comfortable topic of the "virus" that he adamantly hoped or feared had brought about his illness.

Over many weeks of treatment, the therapist repeatedly told the family that she believed Mr. T's symptoms were emotionally based. Gradually, the subject of Mr. T's anger at his parents for their lack of understanding of his "emotions" emerged—as did their ability to express their rage and disappointment with Mr. T for his extreme neediness and the way he had disrupted their lives. Eventually, Mr. T and his parents all agreed to allow him to attend therapy sessions alone.

After 6 months of treatment, Mr. T was able to come to his therapist's office by himself. He also reenrolled in a local university. Mr. T's panic attacks, which had never been as disabling as his severe agoraphobia and passive negativism, resolved with his agoraphobia. This progress initially centered on his determination to see his therapist regularly, even when his father began to refuse to drive him to sessions.

Phobias That Affect Therapy

In standard psychotherapeutic procedure, the patient comes to the office, is met in the waiting room by the therapist, comes into the office and talks, and leaves at the end of the session. For patients with panic disorder who present with symptoms in addition to panic attacks—such as specific phobias—alterations in the standard procedure may be required. Accommodation of patients' specific needs, when necessary, should always facilitate psychodynamic therapeutic work. As with patients who have phobic companions, therapists should allow patients with additional phobias to enter treatment in whatever manner they can within the limitations of their fears. Here too, a more standard therapeutic arrangement can be a goal of the initial phase of treatment.

Case Example

O (See Chapter 6), a 13-year-old girl with panic disorder and a severe elevator phobia, refused to take the elevator to the therapist's top-floor office. O told her mother that the presence of the elevator might make it impossible for her to be in treatment. Because the stairwell was difficult to locate, the therapist met O in the lobby on her first visit and walked up nine flights of stairs with her. Later, the patient told her mother that she knew that she could work with the therapist "because she was so nice to me and walked me up."

Treatment might never have proceeded without this initial accommodation to the patient's phobic concern. Yet this simple step also created a situation in which O reenacted with the therapist the helpless, dependent relationship she routinely had with her mother. This reenactment would require interpretation to the patient at a later point in the treatment—when O's ability to come to the office was no longer threatened.

The timing of an interpretation is as important as its content. In this case, the therapist chose not to interpret O's passive, dependent fears and controlling rage before walking her up the stairs because the therapist could not yet be certain how accurate the interpretation would be. Moreover, the therapist was not sure that O would be able to accept such ideas about herself; the therapist concluded that, having never met the therapist before, O would be unlikely to tolerate any interpretation.

Appropriate therapeutic accommodations may depend on the patient's age and situation in life. For example, young adolescents need to have their parents involved in some way in psychotherapy. For these patients, explanatory meetings with parents are essential at the beginning of treatment, as is regular contact during the course of psychotherapy. Older adolescents, however, often can handle treatment without much parental involvement, in a model resembling psychotherapy with adults.

Countertransference

Patients with panic disorder commonly elicit particular countertransference reactions in therapists who work with them. Most notably, the therapist may avoid pursuing the sources of the patient's anxiety, believing that the patient cannot tolerate the intense anxiety that would attend the exploratory process. Thus, the patient's fear may have a contagious quality.

Case Example

Mr. L (see Chapters 5 and 8) frequently said that he "didn't want to know" a variety of things about which he could easily obtain information. He believed he would become "totally freaked out and go crazy" if the material he discovered was upsetting. Indeed, Mr. L expected everything to upset him; he fantasized about the selfish and sadistic ulterior motives of everyone with whom he came into contact as an explanation for things he might wonder about. He connected these fantasies with the intense disorganization and emotional upheaval he had experienced when he had discovered and viewed his father's video library of sadistic pornography. To guard against the possibility that this compelling fantasy might come true, Mr. L kept himself in a state of extreme ignorance about the way things function, including many simple things, such as how to register for classes in school.

In treatment, Mr. L often was similarly frightened about what his psychiatrist might say to him. At times, Mr. L's terror affected the therapist's comfort in exploring the issues he brought to sessions. The following exchange occurred in the fifth month of psychotherapy.

Patient: I'm really scared to tell you about this because I'm worried we'll have to talk about it, but there's this thing that keeps coming to my mind that I'm worried about.

Therapist: You're putting me in a difficult position. If I ask you about this thing—whatever it is—that you clearly think is important, you're telling me that I'll scare you.

Patient: Yeah, I know. [*Very long silence*] Well, I guess I'll tell you; I'm supposed to be here for you to help me. I have this image; I don't know if it's a memory or not. I'm a kid, like 8 years old, sitting in a dark theater between two adults. I think they're men. One of them is playing with my penis. That's it. I think of that image all the time, but I don't know if it really happened to me or not, or whether it's just from something I heard. Maybe it's a part of the show *A Chorus Line*, and I heard it, and what I'm picturing is actually me in the theater. I just don't know. I can't imagine how it could really have happened to me—What'd you say?

Therapist: I didn't say anything. You seem nervous about what I'll say.

Patient: I am. I'm terrified you'll tell me it really happened and that I'll be a basket case forever and doomed to a life of misery.

Therapist: I do wonder why you always assume that you'll be doomed for the rest of your life.

Mr. L's fantasy/history of sexual abuse by two men—whether real or imagined—clearly was important and formative. Yet although Mr. L provided the therapist with a good opportunity to pursue this image, the therapist refrained from exploring it at that time, consciously believing that it would make the patient too anxious. In fact, crucial material about Mr. L's history of sexual abuse did not emerge again for the better part of a year of psychotherapy.

In the treatment of patients with panic disorder, the therapist and the patient may collude in avoiding more threatening material. The therapist thus becomes de-skilled in the task of uncovering the underlying meaning of panic symptoms. Pursuing frightening fantasies often increases patient anxiety at first; nevertheless, it is the most effective way to bring about significant relief from these symptoms.

Case Example

In the case of Ms. K (see Chapters 5, 6, and 7), the therapist initially responded to the patient's intense fear of her anger with intellectualization and an attempt to water down her expressions of rage. The therapist made nonspecific references to Ms. K's fear of her anger rather than directly noting the fact that she was enraged at the therapist and her mother. Nonetheless, the work steadily progressed, and the patient more directly stated her conflicted wish to kill her mother. Being able to identify her thought/feeling constellation brought Ms. K tremendous relief and significantly diminished her anxiety.

Panic Patients With Borderline Personality Organization

In its description of panic disorder, DSM-IV (American Psychiatric Association 1994) focuses on a specific constellation of symptoms. Yet despite the usefulness of this approach—particularly its specificity—in the classification of patients, large areas of clinical variation remain among patients who meet symptomatic criteria for panic disorder. These crucial differences necessarily affect the usefulness of particular treatment techniques, as well as the nature of the transference that any particular patient forms.

Descriptive psychiatry tends to highlight comorbid psychiatric conditions as a way to describe routine individual differences among patients. From a psychodynamic perspective, however, attention to personality organization (partially described in DSM-IV on Axis II) best portrays broad differences among patients with panic disorder.

The diagnosis of panic disorder, like all of the anxiety disorders described in DSM-IV, does not carry any specificity about the patient's level of personality organization. As such, the diagnosis can apply to patients with a tremendous variety of interpersonal functioning and integrative capacities. Disorganized schizophrenic patients, for example, may meet DSM-IV criteria for panic disorder—as can patients with borderline or neurotic character structures.

A full description of the differences between patients with borderline personality organization and patients with neurotic character structure is beyond the scope of this book (see Kernberg et al. 1989). Nevertheless, because borderline and neurotic patients regularly present for treatment of panic disorder, psychodynamic clinicians must be able to conduct psychotherapy with patients who have either of these diagnoses.

Panic-focused psychodynamic psychotherapy (PFPP), as described in this book, does not require significant modification for patients with less severe personality disorders. With regard to patients with borderline personality organization, however, the nature of transference that the patient forms and the types of interventions that can be helpful at a given time do require some modification of PFPP.

Patients who function at a borderline personality organization level exhibit more distortions in their relationship to reality than neurotic patients. At times, magical ideas are more compelling and harder for these patients to ignore; affective states can be overwhelming. Borderline patients with frequent panic attacks often have more difficulty gaining distance and perspective regarding the frightening, magical thoughts accompanying panic episodes. Therapists must spend a greater amount of time in treatment uncovering persistent, magical beliefs with these patients than in the same endeavor with neurotic patients. For this reason, patients with severe character pathology often require longer-term treatment to address their vulnerability to panic recurrence than neurotic patients.

Borderline and neurotic patients with panic disorder exhibit their most characteristic differences in the relationship they form with the therapist. Both types of panic patients regularly feel as though they depend on the therapist; both can be expected to react to separations during the course of treatment. In contrast to neurotic patients, however, some patients with borderline character structure have difficulty forming a real attachment to the therapist as an individual person. Consequently, they may not engage in the process of psychotherapy as completely as patients who function on a neurotic level.

Patients with borderline personality organization often are frightened and prone to panic when they are alone or when they sense that they are "alone with their problems." These patients desperately want someone to be available to help them. Unfortunately, they may frantically and indiscriminately try to get help and company from many people at once. Relationships often seem shallow and interchangeable for these patients, and therapists may find that the relationships these patients develop in treatment are somewhat empty: Although a borderline patient may initially act as though he or she is extremely intimate with the therapist, the relationship often fails to deepen in an expected manner as the patient spends more time with the therapist. This observation can be extremely useful in gathering information about the quality of the patient's extra-therapeutic relationships. The interchangeability of other relationships with the patient's relationship with the therapist can considerably diminish the impact of treatment.

The therapist therefore must evaluate the patient's characterological makeup during the assessment and planning phases of treatment. Patients with panic disorder and borderline character structure require treatment that focuses not only on their panic symptoms but also on their capacity to tolerate ambivalent feelings and intimacy with others (Kernberg et al. 1989). In the psychotherapeutic approach to these patients, the therapist must address the patient's indiscriminate attachment to people early in treatment.

Case Example

Ms. U, a 35-year-old woman, presented for treatment of panic disorder at a time of extreme emotional crisis when she had just been diagnosed with a life-threatening medical illness. Ms. U had contacted the therapist by telephone several times in the 2 weeks before presentation but had never called back after the therapist returned her calls. In their first telephone contact, Ms. U asked for an emergency appointment with the therapist and told the therapist at great length about her illness.

When Ms. U came to see the therapist the following day, she began her first session by partially disrobing to show the therapist her medical lesion. Ms. U spoke in a pressured manner, describing her anger at her mother and her fear of her panic attacks. She was tearful and extremely difficult to interrupt, even to ask a question. The following dialogue took place within the first 20 minutes of the first interview:

Patient: I really like you; I'm glad I came to see you.

Therapist: Since we just met, and I've hardly said a word, I wonder what you're responding to.

Patient: Well, you're a woman, and you're young. You understand me. I hate—absolutely hate—men. I know it's a problem because I still sometimes think I want to get married some day. What a joke. Since I got sick, it's really gotten extreme. I think men are disgusting; they've enslaved women. This is a sick society. I'm only going to see women doctors now that I'm sick. I blame a lot of my problems on this.

Therapist: So you feel more comfortable with me because I'm a woman.

Patient: It's not only that. It's weird. I feel like I've known you forever. I guess I really don't know anything about you, but it's the way I feel.

Therapist: Maybe it was scary to come and meet a brand new doctor, particularly at a time like this, and it would be less scary if we'd known each other forever.

Patient: What a weird idea. Maybe.

Thus, the therapist begins to focus immediately—during the first session—on the patient's indiscriminate way of relating to the therapist. The therapist's comment that Ms. U's anxiety about meeting her motivates her desire to have "known [the therapist] forever" begins to educate the patient about the magical defenses she uses to ward off intolerable affects.

Panic patients with narcissistic personality disorder also may require special modifications in treatment approach. These patients often experience particularly strong feelings of humiliation about panic symptoms (see Chapter 4). For example, one agoraphobic patient of ours avoided certain situations because he feared that his anxiety would prevent him from performing at his best. For these patients, relatively minor slights can trigger panic episodes, accompanied by rage. Therefore, self-esteem vulnerability becomes intertwined with triggers for panic attacks.

Therapists therefore must assess narcissistic personality traits during the evaluation of patients with panic disorder and account for these traits in conducting psychotherapy. With a narcissistic patient, the therapist should focus immediately on how weak and prone to injury the patient feels—and how these traits contribute to the patient's sense of mounting terror during panic episodes.

Case Example

Mr. V, a 25-year-old unmarried man, described a pattern of recurring panic attacks in the context of rejection by women. In treatment, a pattern emerged: as Mr. V became closer to women, and his romantic relationships evolved, he became increasingly demanding of their attention. He perceived any failure by these women to respond immediately to his needs as a painful rejection. Often, these women pulled back when he began to feel hurt and rejected, which intensified his feelings of rejection, anger, and anxiety. Mr. V's anxiety escalated into panic attacks as these situations evolved into repeated rejections. During his panic episodes, Mr. V was enraged with his girlfriends.

Not surprisingly, this pattern materialized in Mr. V's relationship with his therapist as well. Mr. V frequently missed sessions and felt enraged and injured by the idea of being charged for the missed time. He frequently requested time changes and became furious if alternative times were not available. In the course of psychotherapy, the patient gradually began to recognize these patterns.

Therapist: What do you think happens when you get closer to these women?

Patient: I'm not sure. I feel they are going to abandon me. I really don't trust them. And I feel that you're going to do the same thing.

Therapist: How do you mean?

Patient: That you'll get sick of me. You won't want to be with me anymore. Maybe if you treated me in a nicer or more special way, I wouldn't feel that way.

Therapist: You mean like the requests you make of your girlfriends.

Patient: Yes. And they never do enough. They never measure up.

Thus, Mr. V was beginning to recognize, relatively early in treatment, that his sense of needing special attention from women and his consequent demands were connected with feelings of low self-esteem and fears of abandonment. More work in psychotherapy enabled Mr. V to gain an understanding of the origins of some of these feelings. For example, he reported that his mother suddenly became angry at him and then frequently withdrew and refused to speak to him for days. In one session, Mr. V experienced a panic episode just before a longer-than-usual break in therapy.

Patient: I'm afraid to let you know that I need you. Then you can just hurt me more.

Therapist: What would I do?

Patient: Just leave me. Not respond if I called you. I would get desperate. I remember how terrified I was when my mother began to get angry, realizing that I'd be alone for days. How could she do this to me?

Over the course of 6 months of treatment, Mr. V came to realize that his terror of losing women caused him to be demanding, leading them to withdraw. As he began to acknowledge these fears and his attendant need to be treated as special, his relationships became longer lasting, and his panic episodes resolved.

Panic Patients With Psychotic Disorders

Psychotic patients with panic disorder may suffer acutely as a result of their comorbid panic disorder, and their panic symptoms may become the primary focus of treatment for a time. Although dynamic techniques can help these patients in negotiating their relationship to reality and appreciating the affective triggers that precede their panic attacks, the mainstay of treatment for such patients is necessarily pharmacological, and the central psychotherapeutic focus is the issue of reality testing. Therefore, we do not recommend PFPP for patients with psychosis who also have panic disorder.

Chapter 10

Combining Panic-Focused Psychodynamic Psychotherapy With Other Treatment Approaches

Therapists treating patients with panic disorder can combine psychodynamic psychotherapy with other types of approaches. In particular, psychodynamic knowledge and techniques often can be beneficial in conjunction with cognitive-behavioral treatment or pharmacotherapy.

Psychodynamic Psychotherapy and Cognitive-Behavioral Therapy

Important dynamic factors often underlie a patient's inability to perform particular behavioral tasks; psychodynamic techniques can help the therapist explore these issues. For example, many analysts—beginning with Freud—have used exposure techniques to help patients master fears. Thus, a therapist can add a behavioral component to insight-oriented psychotherapy to provide a particular focus on a specific, bothersome symptom. In addition, cognitive-behavioral interventions often provide important information that facilitates psychodynamic understanding. The following case example illustrates how these two approaches, used together, can help patients rid themselves of some of their anxiety symptoms.

Case Example

Ms. W, a 27-year-old single woman with a long history of panic and agoraphobia, would not go into elevators or airplanes and frequently had panic attacks on the subway. Ms. W's symptoms were so severe that she had to work in a job on the first floor of a building and was afraid to live apart from her mother. She also could not visit her father, who lived in another country.

During her recurrent panic attacks, Ms. W feared that she would not be able to escape the elevator or subway car in which she was traveling. She imagined that if she were stuck, she would not have enough air to breathe, and she would suffocate. She would begin to tear at her face, remove any extra clothing she was wearing, and then grab other people. She thought that knocking herself out would relieve her distress.

Ms. W had some interest in exploring why she had these problems; primarily, however, she wanted to confront the symptoms directly. She noted that she had problems in many other areas in her life that she wanted to address. For example, she had trouble pursuing a more ambitious career because she felt that the demands would be too great, and she avoided relationships with men because she began to feel trapped any time she became close to a man.

Ms. W described a history of upheaval within her family. Her father was an alcoholic who had been cold when sober and shifted between friendliness, criticism, and violence when intoxicated. Ms. W described her mother as temperamental: alternately abandoning and desperately clinging to her daughter. After living in conflict, Ms. W's parents ultimately divorced.

When Ms. W entered treatment, she felt trapped by her mother, but she also felt that she was unable to live alone. She believed that her mother would be terribly hurt if she moved out. Ms. W's mother accused her of siding with her father, although Ms. W did not believe she had. After making these accusations, Ms. W's mother would refuse to speak with her for extended periods of time. Even when Ms. W and her mother were getting along better, however, her mother frequently felt suddenly rejected, saying that Ms. W didn't care about her.

Ms. W admitted that she hated her mother, but then she became anxious about having criticized her mother to the therapist. "Do I sound like a terrible person?" she asked. When Ms. W and her mother were fighting, Ms. W would scratch at her face, similar to the way she did during panic attacks.

Ms. W reported having had multiple surgeries during her childhood for a knee injury; she recalled the anesthesia with terror. She had been terribly frightened when the mask was placed over her face. She preferred not to discuss the experience in more depth.

As part of Ms. W's treatment, the therapist suggested that Ms. W and the therapist ride the elevator together. When they first attempted this exposure technique, Ms. W was terribly frightened and refused to take the elevator to another floor. When returning to the office, the therapist asked Ms. W about her experience.

Therapist: Can you tell me something about what scared you about going on the elevator?

Patient: Yes. I'm simply too frightened, and I'm really all alone in there. What if I got stuck?

Therapist: But I was in there with you. If we were stuck I would help you get out.

Patient: I don't feel that way. I feel completely alone. I don't feel that you would help me.

Therapist: Does this bring anything to mind?

Patient: Well, during my surgeries, I couldn't believe that no one would stop them from putting the anesthesia mask over my face. I thought maybe my mother would do something, but she didn't. I think many times she wasn't even in the room.

Therapist: It's hard for you to believe that I would really help you if we got stuck.

Patient: Yes. I still feel alone.

Shortly thereafter, the patient and the therapist returned to the elevator. This time, Ms. W rode the elevator with the therapist; she was ecstatic about her progress.

Further exploration revealed many particulars that connected Ms. W's panic episodes to her anesthesia experiences. For example, during her panic attacks, Ms. W tore at her face at exactly the position where the anesthesia mask fit over her face. In addition, Ms. W's sense that there was not enough air seemed to relate to her childhood belief that there was inadequate air in the mask and that she would suffocate; the value of being "knocked out" when she was anxious related to the relief she had anticipated when the anesthesia took effect.

A few sessions later, Ms. W described a dream. In the dream, she missed her psychotherapy appointment because she was meeting with an architect who was expanding her office. She had simply forgotten her appointment, but the therapist called and told her that he knew that she had missed the session purposely; Ms. W then came to her appointment. The dream's scene then changed: Ms. W took a 45-minute drive to an amusement park. She enjoyed the rides, which resembled a cartoon about superheroes that she had watched with her nephew.

Ms. W told the therapist that she thought the first scene in the dream referred to an attempt to change her external space rather than deal with what was going on inside of her. She felt that she had accepted that she could not understand her life problems with behavioral treatment alone. Ms. W said that in her dream, she had felt accused by the therapist for missing her therapy session. She also described a sense of pressure to ride more elevators outside of the therapist's office and felt bad that she had not done so.

Ms. W recalled that her father became accusatory when he was drunk; when he was sober, he demanded high levels of academic achievement. He gave quizzes on questions of knowledge that she had trouble answering, which made her feel bad about herself. The therapist then pursued Ms. W's distress regarding the lack of further progress in her behavioral efforts.

Therapist: Can you tell me more about your concern about not going on elevators?

Patient: Yes. I really feel that I have to push ahead with the program. Otherwise I'm not doing anything, and I'm failing. I may not even try going on the elevator, because if I can't, I'll feel I'm back at square one.

Therapist: Has this affected your ability to get on elevators?

Patient: Yes. I feel I don't want to try because I might fail.

Therapist: Do you have a sense of where this kind of pressure arises from?

Patient: Well, I've never really realized that I'm that harsh on myself. It sounds like my father pressuring me to do my work, which I hated. But I've never really thought about it that way.

This realization of intense self-criticism subsequently helped Ms. W take further behavioral steps with less anxiety.

In association to the second part of her dream, Ms. W noted that she had enjoyed the way the superheroes in the cartoon she had watched with her nephew faced and overcame many dangers.

The therapist then pointed out that the length of the drive to the amusement park—45 minutes—was the same as the length of time in Ms. W's psychotherapy sessions. Ms. W was struck by this coincidence; she recalled that she had viewed the elevator as a ride. Ms. W also remembered that when her father was friendly, he would take the family to amusement parks, which she had enjoyed. Subsequent sessions revealed that Ms. W's feelings of excitement and terror with her father—which she reexperienced in the transference—were conflicted, adding to the highly charged nature of her phobia.

Psychodynamic Psychotherapy and Pharmacotherapy

A significant amount of literature describes the benefits of medication in many psychotherapeutic treatments (Beitman and Klerman 1991; Busch and Auchincloss, 1995; Goldhamer 1983; Gutheil 1978, 1982; Kahn 1990; Roose 1990; Shader and Greenblatt 1982). These clinicians and investigators also discussed the importance of the meanings of medications to patients and addressed how to incorporate an understanding of these meanings into psychotherapeutic and psychopharmacological treatments.

Medication can have a modulating effect on intense forms of anxiety that might otherwise prevent a patient from participating in psychodynamic exploration. Therapists should consider medication in treatment recommendations in cases in which a patient's basic professional/school function becomes impossible because of overwhelming panic. Medication also is indicated when a patient presents a significant suicide risk in connection with his or her panic. In many instances, medication is required for only a brief period of time, while the patient is engaged in psychotherapy—at which point a gradual reduction becomes possible.

Chapter 11

Case Example: Ms. P

In this chapter, we review a case example that demonstrates the full course of long-term psychodynamic psychotherapy for a panic patient. The course of treatment follows the outline in Chapter 1. The therapist initially focuses on the circumstances and feelings surrounding panic onset; the therapist then elucidates the dynamic underpinnings of the disorder. As the patient's panic symptoms resolve, the therapist and the patient address the patient's panic vulnerability by working through dynamic conflicts in the transference.

Phase I

Initial Evaluation

Ms. P, a 24-year-old nursing student, presented with the acute onset of panic disorder during her first semester of nursing school. A native of a distant city who had never lived away from her hometown before, Ms. P felt lonely and overwhelmed in her new city. She missed her home and family and constantly compared herself unfavorably with the natives of the city whom she met in nursing school. Although Ms. P had been a straight-A student at a nationally acclaimed college, she felt stupid and inept in nursing school; for the first time in her life, she had difficulty studying.

As Ms. P's first set of exams approached, she began to have panic attacks while studying, with prominent symptoms of shortness of breath, tachycardia, dizziness, and a sensation that she was sweating and "burning up all over." During Ms. P's first panic attack, which occurred while she was alone in her room attempting to study, she became so frightened that she was "ill and dying" that she ran hysterically into a girlfriend's room, crying and demanding to be cared for.

In the ensuing week (before presenting for treatment), Ms. P had several panic attacks in a variety of different settings, although most occurred while she was alone. She continued to fear for her health, particularly during the panic attacks, even though she sensed that her symptoms were "probably emotional." She stopped studying, and she awaited her exams with the hopeless conviction that she would fail and have to leave graduate school, never to achieve her professional goals.

At this point, Ms. P was referred for psychiatric evaluation. She did not want to take medication or participate in behavioral treatment; the psychiatrist recommended twice weekly psychodynamic psychotherapy.

Early Sessions: Circumstances and Feelings Surrounding Panic Onset

Ms. P's therapist first focused on determining in more detail the circumstances preceding panic onset. The therapist discovered that the loneliness and isolation that Ms. P had felt at nursing school had been present for many years. Ms. P felt that her entrance into nursing school signified that she had outachieved her two older sisters. Furthermore, she had imagined that she would be independent and free, with many new friends, and that she could escape what she viewed as her "loser" family. To Ms. P's surprise, however, she missed her family terribly at school; she also felt unable to establish relationships with the new people she met, which intensified her feelings of loneliness and isolation. Ms. P felt that she could not fit in with other people and that "the weirdness of my family" had permeated her personality, making her a social misfit.

From this information, the therapist hypothesized that Ms. P's panic onset related, in part, to her feelings of loneliness and loss. The therapist then explored the origins of these feelings further with Ms. P.

Ms. P apparently had struggled with feelings of loneliness since the death of her mother 7 years earlier. Her difficulties with this loss were evident even in the first session: she became tearful almost immediately when she told her therapist about her mother's death.

Yet when the therapist reflected that she clearly was still quite upset about the loss, Ms. P suddenly and seemingly unaccountably became angry, accusing the therapist of "using stupid, hokey shrink formulas. . . . It's just too neat. 'Poor baby, never recovered from the loss of her mother,'" she said in a mocking tone, adding, "That is total bullshit."

Additional exploration of Ms. P's experience of her mother's death provided further evidence, however, of her difficulty in managing the loss. Ms. P's mother had been diagnosed with cancer when Ms. P was 12 years old; despite numerous surgical interventions and chemotherapy, she died (at home) when Ms. P was 17 years old. Thus, Ms. P grew up in a household in which the threat of death was imminent for a long period of time. Ms. P's entire family handled this threat with dense denial, however, treating her mother's illness as an unmentionable subject. Even on her deathbed, emaciated and feverish, Ms. P's mother told her daughter that she would be better soon. Ms. P desperately wanted to believe her mother's reassurances about her health and about everything else, such as Ms. P's chronic fears that she would always be unpopular.

After her mother died, Ms. P felt "shattered" and surprised, despite the fact that she had been acquainted with her mother's medical diagnosis for years. Ms. P had denied the significance of the illness to herself. After her mother died, she felt that her whole life was coming apart, and she spent as much time as possible at her older sister's house; she consciously thought of this sister as "another mother." Despite these efforts, however, Ms. P's intense feelings of loss and loneliness persisted.

This information enabled both the therapist and the patient to gain a clearer understanding of the immediate precipitants of Ms. P's panic attacks. At the time of her panic onset, for example, Ms. P was studying something that she consciously connected with the cause of her mother's death. Ms. P also realized that when she completed graduate school, she would be in a position to act in a caring capacity for people like her mother. During the course of these discussions, Ms. P also revealed that her mother, during her final illness, had been "burning up with fever"—a symptom Ms. P herself reexperienced during her panic episodes.

Formulation of Dynamic Issues

The therapist continued to explore the thoughts Ms. P had at the times of her panic attacks. Ms. P gradually revealed that she lived with a constant, pervasive, barely conscious fantasy that her dead mother was observing her. This fantasy began to emerge when Ms. P spoke about needing to listen to her Walkman® when she studied alone in her room because "the silence of there being no one else there with me is deafening; I need to distract myself." As Ms. P performed her daily activities at school, even as she crossed the street, she found herself thinking, "If Mommy could see me now, she'd see. . . ."

Ms. P pictured a "powerful, somewhat critical force or person" observing her from on high; she imagined that this individual would be extremely impressed with her accomplishments, just as she would have wanted her mother to be. (Although Ms. P had converted to Catholicism to be like her sister, who had converted after their mother's death, she was not religious and she did not believe in God).

Ms. P often found these fantasies that she was being observed quite gratifying; they tended to emphasize romantic ways in which she would have liked to picture herself "in my new life: all grown up and sophisticated, living alone in New York [or] in a fancy graduate school." However, Ms. P experienced panic attacks when this fantasy seemed most unrealistic and unrewarding and she felt most alone without her mother. Studying the illness that her mother died from, realizing that she would care for people like her mother, and feeling the absence of her family brought Ms. P's own loneliness and isolation into clear focus for her and shattered her fantasy. Ms. P's panic symptoms themselves, including fantasied threats of her own impending death, represented an unconscious recognition of her mother's death as well as an identification with her sick, hopeless mother.

Ms. P's panic attacks resolved completely—never to return—after 6 weeks of twice weekly psychotherapy. Specifically, her symptoms disappeared after a session in which the therapist interpreted how devastating the loss of this fantasy, and her mother, were to Ms. P. She responded to this interpretation with interest and embarrassment. She felt that her attachment to her mother was "immature"—yet another type of behavior that demonstrated what a "baby" she was.

Although Ms. P's panic attacks ceased relatively rapidly after the beginning of her psychotherapy, she remained extremely insecure socially. This social anxiety had been present since her childhood, and further exploration of this anxiety provided greater insight into the origins of her panic.

Ms. P gradually became aware of her extreme dependence on her mother's presence throughout her childhood (something she had adamantly denied when she began psychotherapy). Ms. P had always been worried as a child; even before her mother became ill, she had been particularly anxious about being separated from her mother, even briefly.

Ms. P also felt that she had to compete with her sisters to gain the attention she sought from her mother. Ms. P was the youngest of three girls in her family (8 years younger than her next older sister). She had always been unpopular, and she preferred to stay at home with her mother rather than develop relationships with her peers. In Ms. P's mind, she strove to be academically successful in an attempt to gain her mother's approval. She wanted to prove to her mother that she was "the best" of the three sisters. Although she was, in fact, more academically successful than her sisters, she felt that she never got what she sought from her mother.

In addition to these efforts to be academically successful, Ms. P began to recognize that she had used—without realizing it—other means of obtaining her mother's attention, as well as the attention of other persons. For example, she experienced and communicated an urgent neediness, expressed by relentless self-deprecation and advertisement about how helpless and incapable she felt she was. When Ms. P was a child, her older sisters became enraged with her when she behaved in this needy and demanding way with their mother.

Over several months of psychotherapy, Ms. P appeared to be highly conflicted about her aggressive wishes to outdo her sisters in search of her mother's attention. By emphasizing her incapacities, she denied these aggressive wishes to herself; she also punished herself for these wishes via self-denigration. This behavior enabled her to continue to compete aggressively with her sisters.

At the time of Ms. P's panic onset, her aggressive, competitive attempts to symbolically obtain her mother's attention and approval were even more threatening than usual: graduate school was quite competitive, and it represented even greater success than she had achieved before. Thus, Ms. P's panic attacks served as self-punishment for her aggressive desire to outachieve her sisters.

Phase 2

Addressing Conflicts in the Transference

Focusing on the transference enabled the therapist to elucidate and address characterological underpinnings to Ms. P's persistent social anxiety and vulnerability to panic attacks. Thus, despite Ms. P's rapid symptomatic improvement, she remained extremely dependent on her therapist. Ms. P's symptoms appeared to resolve in part because her therapist had become a replacement figure for her mother; Ms. P again felt that an older woman was caring for her. Ms. P admired her therapist; indeed, she idealized her therapist, describing the therapist as "brilliant, beautiful, and perfect"—much as she had idealized her mother when her mother was alive—and comparing herself unfavorably with her therapist in all ways. Yet Ms. P acknowledged her therapist's point that she had set up a fantasied representation of the therapist that corresponded to her idea of her mother. Ms. P deeply longed for praise; she also felt underappreciated by her therapist, as she had by her mother.

Using information gleaned from exploring this transference, the therapist and the patient recognized that Ms. P routinely set up relationships with other women in which she felt inferior and unable to compete, particularly with regard to the attention of men. Consequently, she became enraged and resentful toward these women. Ms. P directed most of her conscious energy toward women she admired for their social prowess, whom she wanted to have as friends. Yet she frequently felt that these women were neglecting and hurting her because they did not pay enough attention to her.

Thus, Ms. P seemed to be living out a fantasy in these relationships: "See what I've given up for you (any hope or fantasy of a romance of my own), and you don't even appreciate it!" In the course of psychotherapy, Ms. P gradually realized that this set of ideas had been pervasive in her relationship with her mother and older sisters and that it continued to be a central aspect of her relationship with her therapist.

Ms. P initially tried to ignore the therapist's comments about the manifestations of this state of affairs in the transference; she acted as if any open acknowledgment of her feelings would somehow threaten her relationship with her therapist. Eventually, however, Ms. P began to understand that she feared her anger and worried that her neediness would drive the therapist away. The therapist helped Ms. P recognize these previously unconscious dangers and explore them in the "safe" atmosphere of therapy, and Ms. P gained the conviction that such feelings would not lead to catastrophic loss.

Over time, Ms. P developed an increased ability to recognize and think about the unconscious fantasies she enacted repeatedly. She also gained more self-confidence, and she stopped setting up relationships along this pattern. As she became less anxious about her performance, she gradually—haltingly—began to establish romantic relationships with men.

Working Through

Further efforts to work through Ms. P's characterological vulnerability to panic addressed her avoidance of involvements with men. For example, Ms. P complained about feeling "incomplete as a person"; she explained that because of her long history of severe separation anxiety and unwillingness to leave her mother's side, she had missed crucial normative developmental experiences, such as attending her high school prom. Missing these experiences greatly humiliated her.

Consequently, Ms. P felt that she could not compete with female peers in the adult sexual world. She thought of herself as "not really a woman, more of a child or a neuter," yet she desperately longed to be more mature and to have a romantic life with men. Ms. P articulated this set of fantasies most clearly in the middle of her second year of graduate school: during a school lecture about female sexuality, she revealed, she found herself musing that she ought to donate her own sexual organs to another woman who could actually make use of them—as Ms. P was doomed never to do. These thoughts made her feel miserable and profoundly humiliated. Nevertheless, Ms. P's understanding of her need to set up relationships in which she felt inferior and unable to compete, particularly as explored in the transference, helped her feel safer competing with other women for the attention of men.

Ms. P gained further understanding of her need to abnegate herself in her relationships with men and women when she was able to comprehend the significance of a series of memories that arose during the second year of her treatment. Ms. P had been discussing her older sisters' meanness to her and how "weird" she had been as a child. She said that even when she was an adolescent, her mother had described Ms. P to her friends as "different, my little baby." "That's because I was so much younger than my sisters," Ms. P said.

When the therapist asked Ms. P about her understanding of why she was that much younger than her sisters, Ms. P initially was at a loss to explain the age difference. Over the course of several sessions, however, Ms. P began to remember things that her sisters, her father, and family friends had said. Although she had always known these things, she had never allowed herself to connect the different pieces of information. Apparently, Ms. P had been an accidental child, conceived after her mother believed herself to be past menopause. Furthermore, Ms. P's mother had attempted to obtain an abortion, which had failed.

As Ms. P made these "discoveries," her own fantasy of giving up everything for her mother gradually made more sense to her: she became aware of the intense and persistent guilt she had always felt in relation to her mother because of the mere fact of her existence as well as her fury with her mother for truly "preferring" her sisters to her. Through this work, Ms. P gradually realized that her submission to powerful women and self-disparagement with regard to men served as self-imposed punishment for burdening her mother. This realization about how her guilt was affecting her helped Ms. P to become less inhibited about asserting herself—without punishing herself—academically and in her relationships with men.

Ms. P has not been in treatment for the past 8 years. A recent follow-up conversation revealed that Ms. P has remained entirely panic-free for 10 years. Although she has been extremely successful in all areas of her life, however, her relations with her family remain strained.

Chapter 12
Conclusion

Psychiatrists have made enormous progress in the treatment of panic disorder and agoraphobia over the past 30 years. In particular, pharmacological and cognitive-behavioral treatments have provided significant inroads toward relief from intense anxiety in many patients. Nevertheless, excitement about these approaches often has been overshadowed by the reality of many patients' continued problems, which include frequent panic recurrence (Ballenger 1991; Noyes et al. 1989b; Pecknold et al. 1988; Rosenbaum 1992) and the chronic characterological problems with which these patients continue to struggle.

Persistent anxiety symptoms can have a profound impact on patients' quality of life (Katon et al. 1992; Markowitz et al. 1989). In this book, we have attempted to define psychodynamic factors in patients with panic disorder that we have found are related to persistent personality problems and panic vulnerability. In addition, we have suggested psychodynamic psychotherapeutic approaches to address these problems.

As we noted in Chapter 10, we believe that cognitive-behavioral and psychopharmacological treatment approaches can be valuable. Psychodynamic approaches often help in cognitive-behavioral treatments; conversely, behavioral efforts can provide important information about ongoing psychodynamic conflicts. Medication also may be a valuable adjunct to psychodynamic exploration: it can help patients discuss the particulars of their fears more easily. Nevertheless, in our experience, panic symptoms resolve rapidly for many patients with psychodynamic psychotherapy alone.

In recent years, many mental health practitioners have regarded psychodynamic approaches as ineffective for specific psychiatric disorders. This attitude probably relates to the tendency of psychodynamic clinicians to shy away from a symptom-focused approach to specific disorders—based on the notion that this style is too directive and therefore can detract from listening to the patient. We believe, however, that symptom-focused treatment can help to provide rapid symptom relief in the same way that medication can. Such therapy, furthermore, need not make further dynamic work, aimed at more chronic characterological problems, more difficult.

Systematic research is needed to ascertain the efficacy of psychodynamic psychotherapy for the treatment of panic disorder; we hope this manual will help to facilitate this process. In the meantime, we believe that the focused psychodynamic approaches suggested in this book can help therapists treating patients with this complex and often disabling illness.

References

Abend S: Psychoanalytic psychotherapy, in Handbook of Phobia Therapy. Edited by Lindeman C. Northvale, NJ, and London: Jason Aronson, 1989, pp 393–403

American Psychiatric Association: Diagnostic and Statistical Manual of Mental Disorders, 3rd Edition, Revised. Washington, DC, American Psychiatric Association, 1987

American Psychiatric Association: Diagnostic and Statistical Manual of Mental Disorders, 4th Edition. Washington, DC, American Psychiatric Association, 1994

Andrews G, Pollock C, Stewart G: The determination of defense style by questionnaire. Arch Gen Psychiatry 46:455–460, 1989

Andrews G, Stewart G, Morris-Yates A, et al: Evidence for a general neurotic syndrome. Br J Psychiatry 157:6–12, 1990

Arrindell W, Emmelkamp PMG, Monsma A, et al: The role of perceived parental rearing practices in the etiology of phobic disorders: a controlled study. Br J Psychiatry 143:183–187, 1983

Ballenger JC: Long-term pharmacologic treatment of panic disorder. J Clin Psychiatry 52(suppl 2):18–23, 1991

Beck AT, Sokol L, Clark DA, et al: A crossover study of focused cognitive therapy of panic disorder. Am J Psychiatry 149:778–783, 1992

Beitman BD, Klerman GL (eds): Integrating Pharmacotherapy and Psychotherapy. Washington, DC, American Psychiatric Press, 1991

Bibring E: Psychoanalysis and the dynamic psychotherapies. J Am Psychoanal Assoc 2:745–770, 1954

Busch FN, Auchincloss E: The psychology of prescribing and taking medication, in Psychodynamic Concepts in General Psychiatry. Edited by Schwartz H. Washington, DC, American Psychiatric Press, 1995, pp 401–416

Busch FN, Cooper AM, Klerman GL, et al: Neurophysiological, cognitive-behavioral, and psychoanalytic approaches to panic disorder: toward an integration. Psychoanalytic Inquiry 11: 316–332, 1991

Busch FN, Shear MK, Cooper AM, et al: An empirical study of defense mechanisms in panic disorder. J Nerv Ment Dis 183: 299–303, 1995

Craske MG: Cognitive behavioral treatment of panic, in American Psychiatric Press Review of Psychiatry, Vol 7. Edited by Frances AJ, Hales RE. Washington, DC, American Psychiatric Press, 1988, pp 121–137

Craske MG, Brown TA, Barlow DH: Behavioral treatment of panic: a two-year follow-up. Behavioral Therapy 22:289–304, 1991

Deutsch H: The genesis of agoraphobia. Int J Psychoanal 10:51–69, 1929

Faravelli C: Life events preceding the onset of panic disorder. J Affect Disord 9:103–105, 1985

Fava M, Anderson K, Rosenbaum JF: Anger attacks: possible variants of panic and major depressive disorders. Am J Psychiatry 147:867–870, 1990

Freud S: On the grounds for detaching a particular syndrome from neurasthenia under the description "anxiety neurosis" (1895), in The Standard Edition of the Complete Psychological Works of Sigmund Freud, Vol 3. Translated and edited by Strachey J. London, Hogarth Press, 1962, pp 87–120

Freud S: The interpretation of dreams (1900), in The Standard Edition of the Complete Psychological Works of Sigmund Freud, Vols 4 and 5. Translated and edited by Strachey J. London, Hogarth Press, 1953, pp xi–751

Freud S: Inhibitions, symptoms and anxiety (1926), in The Standard Edition of the Complete Psychological Works of Sigmund Freud, Vol 20. Translated and edited by Strachey J. London, Hogarth Press, 1950, pp 75–175

Fyer AJ, Liebowitz MR, Gorman JM, et al: Discontinuation of alprazolam treatment in panic patients. Am J Psychiatry 144: 303–308, 1987

George DT, Anderson P, Nutt DJ, et al: Aggressive thoughts and behavior: another symptom of panic disorder? Acta Psychiatr Scand 79:500–502, 1989

Goldhamer PM: Psychotherapy and pharmacotherapy: the challenge of integration. Can J Psychiatry 28:173–177, 1983

Greenson RR: The Technique and Practice of Psychoanalysis, Vol 1. Madison, CT, International Universities Press, 1967

Gutheil TG: Drug therapy: alliance and compliance. Psychosomatics 19:219–225, 1978

Gutheil TG: The psychology of psychopharmacology. Bull Menninger Clin 46:321–330, 1982

Jacobs T: On countertransference reactions. J Am Psychoanal Assoc 34:289–307, 1986

Kagan J, Reznick JS, Snidman N, et al: Origins of panic disorder, in Neurobiology of Panic Disorder. Edited by Ballenger J. New York, Wiley, 1990, pp 71–87

Kahn D: The dichotomy of drugs and psychotherapy, in The Psychiatric Clinics of North America. Edited by Marcus ER. Philadelphia, PA, WB Saunders, 1990, pp 197–208

Katon WJ, Von Korff M, Lin E: Panic disorder: relationship to high medical utilization. Am J Med 92(suppl 1A):75–115, 1992

Kernberg OF, Seltzer MA, Koenigsberg HW, et al: Psychodynamic Psychotherapy of Borderline Patients. New York, Basic Books, 1989

Klein DF: Delineation of two drug-responsive anxiety syndromes. Psychopharmacologia 5:397–408, 1964

Klein DF: False suffocation alarms, spontaneous panics, and related conditions: an integrative hypothesis. Arch Gen Psychiatry 50:306–317, 1993

Klein DF, Gorman JM: A model of panic and agoraphobic development. Acta Psychiatr Scand 76:87–95, 1987

Kleiner L, Marshall WL: The role of interpersonal problems in the development of agoraphobia with panic attacks. Journal of Anxiety Disorders 1:313–323, 1987

Last CG, Barlow DH, O'Brien GT: Precipitants of agoraphobia: role of stressful life events. Psychol Rep 54:567–570, 1984

Leonard HL, Rapoport JL: Anxiety disorders in childhood and adolescence, in American Psychiatric Press Review of Psychiatry, Vol 8. Edited by Tasman A, Hales RE, Frances AJ. Washington, DC, American Psychiatric Press, 1989

Malan DH: Individual Psychotherapy and the Science of Psychodynamics. London, Butterworth, 1979

Mann J: The case of the conquered woman, in Time-Limited Psychotherapy. Cambridge, MA, Harvard University Press, 1973.

Markowitz JS, Weissman MM, Ouellette R, et al: Quality of life in panic disorder. Arch Gen Psychiatry 46:984–992, 1989

Marks IM: Agoraphobic syndrome (phobic anxiety state). Arch Gen Psychiatry 23:538–553, 1970

McGrath PJ, Robinson D, Stewart JW: Atypical panic attacks in major depression (letter). Am J Psychiatry 142:1224, 1985

Milrod BL: The continuing usefulness of psychoanalysis in the treatment of panic disorder. J Am Psychoanal Assoc 43:151–162, 1995

Milrod BL, Busch FN: The long-term outcome of treatments for panic disorder: a review of the literature. J Nerv Ment Dis, in press.

Milrod BL, Shear MK: Dynamic treatment of panic disorder: a review. J Nerv Ment Dis 179:741–743, 1991a

Milrod BL, Shear MK: Psychodynamic treatment of panic: three case histories. Hosp Community Psychiatry 42:311–312, 1991b

Noyes R, Garvey JM, Cook BL: Follow-up study of patients with panic disorder and agoraphobia with panic attacks treated with tricyclic antidepressants. J Affect Disord 16:249–257, 1989a

Noyes R, Garvey JM, Cook BL, et al: Problems with tricyclic use in patients with panic disorder or agoraphobia: results of a naturalistic follow-up study. J Clin Psychiatry 50:163–169, 1989b

Noyes R, Reich J, Christiansen J, et al: Outcome of panic disorder: relationship to diagnostic subtypes and comorbidity. Arch Gen Psychiatry 47:809–818, 1990

Ost LG: Applied relaxation in the treatment of panic disorder. Behav Res Ther 26:13–22, 1988

O'Sullivan G, Marks I: Follow-up studies of behavioral treatment of phobic and obsessive compulsive neurosis. Psychiatric Annals 21:368–373, 1991

Parker G: Reported parental characteristics of agoraphobics and social phobics. Br J Psychiatry 135:555–560, 1979

Parker G, Tupling H, Brown LB: A parental bonding instrument. Br J Med Psychol 52:1–10, 1979

Pecknold JD, Swinson RP, Kuch K, et al: Alprazolam in panic disorder and agoraphobia; results from a multicenter trial, III: discontinuation effects. Arch Gen Psychiatry 45:429–436, 1988

Perris C, Jacobsson L, Lindstrom H, et al: Development of a new inventory for assessing memories of parental rearing behavior. Acta Psychiatr Scand 61:265–274, 1980

Pollock C, Andrews G: Defense styles associated with specific anxiety disorders. Am J Psychiatry 146:1500–1502, 1989

Roose S: The use of medication in combination with psychoanalytic psychotherapy or psychoanalysis, in Psychiatry. Edited by Michels R. New York, Lippincott, 1990, pp 1–8

Rosenbaum JF: Evaluation and management of the treatment-resistant anxiety disorder patient. Bull Menninger Clin 56 (suppl A):50–60, 1992

Rosenbaum JF, Biederman J, Gersten M, et al: Behavioral inhibition in children of parents with panic disorder and agoraphobia. Arch Gen Psychiatry 45:463–470, 1988

Roy-Byrne PP, Geraci M, Uhde TW: Life events and the onset of panic disorder. Am J Psychiatry 143:1424–1427, 1986

Sandler AM: Aspects of the analysis of a neurotic patient. Int J Psychoanal 69:317–326, 1988

Sandler J, Kennedy H, Tyson RL: The Technique of Child Psychoanalysis. Cambridge, MA, Harvard University Press, 1980

Shader RI, Greenblatt DJ: Editorial: Pharmacotherapy and psychotherapy. J Clin Psychopharmacol 2:1, 1982

Shear MK, Cooper AM, Klerman GL, et al: A psychodynamic model of panic disorder. Am J Psychiatry 150:859–866, 1993

Sifneos PE: Short-Term Psychotherapy and Emotional Crisis. Cambridge, MA, Harvard University Press, 1972

Silber A: Panic attacks facilitating recall and mastery: implications for psychoanalytic techniques. J Am Psychoanal Assoc 37: 337–364, 1989

Silove D: Perceived parental characteristics and reports of early parental deprivation in agoraphobic patients. Aust N Z J Psychiatry 20:365–369, 1986

Solyom L, Beck P, Solyom C, et al: Some etiological factors in phobic neurosis. Can Psychiatr Assoc J 19:69–78, 1974

Torgerson S: Childhood and family characteristics in panic and generalized anxiety disorders. Am J Psychiatry 143:630–632, 1986

Tucker WI: Diagnosis and treatment of the phobic reaction. Am J Psychiatry 112:825–830, 1956

Tyrer P: Neurosis divisible? Lancet 92:685–688, 1985

Tyrer P: Classification of anxiety disorders: a critique of DSM-III (discussion paper). J Affect Disord 11:99–104, 1986

Tyrer P, Seivewright N, Ferguson B, et al: The general neurotic syndrome: a coaxial diagnosis of anxiety, depression and personality disorder. Acta Psychiatr Scand 85:201–206, 1992

Viederman M, Perry SW: Use of a psychodynamic life narrative in the treatment of depression in the physically ill. Gen Hosp Psychiatry 3:177–185, 1980

Wade SL, Monroe SM, Michelson LK: Chronic life stress and treatment outcome in agoraphobia with panic attacks. Am J Psychiatry 150:1491–1495, 1993

Weissman MM, Leckman JF, Merikengas KR, et al: Depression and anxiety disorders in parents and children. Arch Gen Psychiatry 41:845–852, 1984

Index

www.ingramcontent.com/pod-product-compliance
Ingram Content Group UK Ltd.
Pitfield, Milton Keynes, MK11 3LW, UK
UKHW021840100926
8556IPUK00014B/935/J

9 780880 488716